Treating Arthritis: The

Julia Davies, BSc (Hons), Dip CNM, is a (
ing at the Margaret Hills Clinic in War
natural treatment of arthritis. The clini(
by Julia's grandmother Margaret Hills,
young child, Julia developed juvenile idiopatnic artnritis and followed the
very same treatment programme she now recommends to many others
seeking to resolve their arthritis. She has had no signs of the condition since
the age of 11 when her last remaining symptoms disappeared. Julia gained
a degree in human physiology, which gave her a scientific understanding of health problems, before completing further training at the College
of Naturopathic Medicine. The Margaret Hills Clinic attracts people with
arthritis from around the globe; many are treated at a distance due to the
difficulties of travel and mobility.

Overcoming Common Problems Series

Selected titles

A full list of titles is available from Sheldon Press,
36 Causton Street, London SW1P 4ST and on our website at
www.sheldonpress.co.uk

Overcoming Common Problems

Treating Arthritis
The supplements guide

JULIA DAVIES

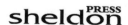

First published in Great Britain in 2012

Sheldon Press
36 Causton Street
London SW1P 4ST
www.sheldonpress.co.uk

The author and publisher have made every effort to ensure that the external website and email addresses included in this book are correct and up to date at the time of going to press. The author and publisher are not responsible for the content, quality or continuing accessibility of the sites.

British Library Cataloguing-in-Publication Data
A catalogue record for this book is available from the British Library

ISBN 978–1–84709–193–2
eBook ISBN 978–1–84709–194–9

Typeset by Caroline Waldron, Wirral, Cheshire
First printed in Great Britain by Ashford Colour Press
Subsequently digitally printed in Great Britain

Produced on paper from sustainable forests

To my grandma,
who taught me that life is 10 per cent what happens to you
and 90 per cent what you choose to do about it

Contents

Preface

My awareness of arthritis began as a child. At the age of eight, I experienced the first symptoms of this painful, debilitating condition. As well as classic joint pain, I had chronic headaches, muscle aches, twisting fingers and nervous twitches and found normal daily activities exhausting, uncomfortable and painful. I was eventually diagnosed with juvenile idiopathic arthritis – idiopathic meaning my doctor didn't know why or how the condition had come about. I was extremely fortunate to have as my grandmother Margaret Hills, who had for her own sake devised a treatment for arthritis using completely natural methods. During her nursing career she had both osteoarthritis and rheumatoid arthritis for which no medical help worked. As a result she used her understanding of the human body, together with many months of research, to eventually rid herself completely of arthritis. The same treatment proved successful for me over a period of about 12 to 18 months, after which time I was completely free from any signs of arthritis. Twenty or so years later, I am in great health and my symptoms have never returned.

Since this early experience, I have devoted my entire life to researching arthritis and natural health so that I can help others to recover from this chronic condition. There is never a time when I don't keep learning: the human body has so many remarkable abilities, it is just a case of finding the means to tap into those resources so that optimal health can be achieved. Keeping abreast of the latest research and putting into practice the new developments enhances my grandmother's natural treatment and gives it increasing credibility as a treatment option for all kinds of health conditions.

In this book my aim is to provide in-depth explanations of natural supplements that may help alleviate arthritis: why they work, how they work and how to incorporate them into your own treatment plan. I will explore the naturopathic perspective on the causes of arthritis and its various natural treatment methods. I will include dietary advice and examples of typical supplement programmes. With all this information to hand, you can start making practical steps towards recovery today. In my view, recovery from arthritis does *not* mean simply controlling the symptoms or masking the pain you experience. My aim is for you to rid yourself completely of any signs and symptoms of arthritis so that your joint problems become nothing more than a distant memory. Your arthritis medications will eventually become unnecessary.

Many people with arthritis feel very isolated. As time goes on, their doctor or consultant may tell them that nothing more can be done other than to go home and learn to live with their condition. Even their families can become frustrated and exasperated – arthritis can affect the whole family, day in, day out, for many years. I often hear people with arthritis say things like, 'People just don't want to hear it; everyone is fed up with me, they don't even ask how I am any more.' Does this sound familiar? If it rings true for you, I want you to know that there *is* another way and it *is* possible to change your situation to achieve good health again.

This book does not aim to disregard current medical strategies in treating arthritis, only to bring to the forefront of people's minds that the *possibilities* are out there now for achieving total resolution of the symptoms of arthritis.

There is no better feeling than taking control of your own health – the satisfaction you will experience once you have achieved complete remission of symptoms is incredible.

Introduction

Arthritis treatments: the current situation

One in five adults in the UK has some form of arthritis. Current medical thinking has highlighted the lack of success in treating this condition with conventional drug regimes. The following quote is taken from the medical journal *Current Drug Targets* (2010) in reference to the available treatments for osteoarthritis:

> It is evident that there is a *great need for the development* [my emphasis] of disease modifying agents in order to improve quality of life as well as to relieve the community of the enormous socio-economic burden of the disease [osteoarthritis].[1]

There isn't currently a great deal on offer for treating arthritis long term other than replacing the joint and masking the symptoms with medication. This may offer a short-term solution for some people, but what about the several millions of others for whom this is not an effective route to follow?

Even if a person is doing well on medication and his or her symptoms are well-controlled, there are still some concerns. Arthritis involves inflammation and damage to the joints and the strong anti-inflammatory medications currently on offer not only suppress inflammation but also prevent crucial repairing of the area. Inflammation is actually one of the body's critical self-protecting systems; it is heightened when there is damaged tissue or infection, but is also a process that aids subsequent repair of that part of the body. In the short term, taking medicines to counter the inflammatory process is often necessary, as otherwise the inflammation can become dangerous. However, we must also think about the long-term effects of interfering with the body's natural ability to repair itself. When taking drugs, the symptoms may be controlled but the disease is still progressing regardless.

There is no simple answer to arthritis; it is an extremely common, yet very complex disease for which the medical profession has so far struggled to find a sustainable solution. Pain and inflammation can sometimes be eased, but over the long term such symptoms generally get worse. Stronger and stronger drugs are needed and your only hope may be to undergo surgery and receive a joint replacement. Such surgery can be very successful, until the arthritis symptoms develop in another joint – when, sadly, the same story begins yet again.

You may have reached the point of intense frustration and that is why you are reading this book, wondering how you can help yourself. I hope that I can help you find the right way forward.

A note on supplements: Research has shown that up to 90 per cent of people with arthritis have tried some form of complementary or alternative medicine. The use of supplements, however, is currently a minefield, with hundreds of brands of essentially the same substance on the market. It takes an expert to distinguish between products and know the correct and appropriate way to use them. The supplements featured in this book, therefore, are those which, in my experience, are the most likely to produce good results.

You will be able to look up an individual supplement by its index entry or simply browse through the book to investigate the many different options available. I recommend that you read the book in its entirety before beginning any treatment as you will see that you need to take more than one action to achieve the results I describe.

Note to the reader

The programme herein is not intended to replace the services of trained health professionals, or be a substitute for medical advice. You are advised to consult with your health professional with regard to matters that may require diagnosis or medical attention.

1

What is arthritis and what might cause it?

Osteoarthritis represents a disease group with disease subsets that have different underlying pathophysiological mechanisms.[1]

In other words, everyone is different! Arthritis is an umbrella term that encompasses over 200 conditions involving the joints, distinguishable by their symptoms and causes. The word arthritis stems from 'arthro', meaning joints, combined with 'itis', meaning inflammation. However, some forms of the condition do not necessarily involve inflammation and are better described as a degenerative breakdown of the joint function due to a variety of factors. Osteoarthritis, which may affect just one or two joints, is considered to be the simple form; it involves a gradual degeneration of joint cartilage, which eventually impairs the function of the joint. Other forms of arthritis may involve severe inflammation, affecting not only the joints but also muscles and even, in some cases, organs of the body such as the heart.

Many different factors, often occurring over a period of years, contribute to the onset of arthritis. These may include poor diet, undue stress, lack of fresh air, environmental factors and emotional issues, to name but a few. In my experience, however, the common theme among people with arthritis is the build-up of acid that crystallizes within the joints and causes pain and injury. All the other issues simply contribute to this acidity level.

The symptoms of arthritis differ greatly from one person to the next and vary hugely in severity. But arthritis is generally considered a progressive disease, meaning it worsens over time. Its responsiveness to drug treatment varies a great deal. So how, given all these variables, can we expect a *single* wonder cure or drug?

A wider, more holistic view is necessary to make any progress. No matter how effective the next new drug is for pain or inflammation, unless it takes into account the differing causes and individual nature of the condition the solution will not be found. I believe that treatment of the condition using naturopathic principles is the way to success. In the next chapter we will look at what that entails. First, though, we need to look at the reasons why people are affected by arthritis, as these need to be understood in order for treatment to be effective.

What is the root cause of arthritis?

There are many theories and opinions as to what causes the onset and progression of arthritic diseases, but so far none of them are particularly conclusive. My experience and understanding supports the theory that joint problems are caused by an excess of acid, both in the whole body and within the joints themselves. Over time, often years, acid accumulates and has a degenerative effect on the joints. Acidity in the tissues of the body causes inflammation and pain. By exploring this theory, we can be clearer about treatment options that aim to reduce and clear out the excess acid.

What does it mean to have too much acid in my body?

The term used when measuring the acidity or alkalinity of a substance is pH. It is a scale ranging from 1 to 14, 1 being extremely acid and 14 being extremely alkaline. Alkali neutralizes acid and vice versa. A neutral pH is simply somewhere in the middle of the two and so can neither be described as acid or alkaline. Water is neutral at pH 7.

The pH level is a crucial aspect of the body's overall balance for healthy living. This healthy balance is referred to as 'homeostasis', which means the ability of the body to adjust its internal environment in order to maintain a stable equilibrium (balance) of critical factors such as body temperature, blood sugar and pH level. Homeostasis is critical to life.

Many diseases, including arthritis, occur as a result of disturbed homeostasis, specifically one that entails a reduced pH level. The resulting excess acid within the body can create all sorts of health problems, such as pain, inflammation and progressive damage to joints. The immune system may also be affected, causing the body to attack its own joints – a condition we know as rheumatoid arthritis.

The pH level is one of the most critical components of homeostatic balance, so it makes sense that restoring pH to its correct level will halt the disease process and gradually relieve the symptoms of the condition.

How does our body pH become out of balance?

Because of the way we live today – our foods, our work pressures and our lifestyles – our body's pH is likely to become more acidic rather than more alkaline. Acid is produced in the following ways:

- from normal metabolism (i.e. within the body itself);
- from dietary sources (i.e. acidic food and drink);
- from stress – both chronic stress and acute periods of stress or trauma;
- from environmental pollutants (e.g. cigarette smoke, exhaust fumes, electro-magnetic pollution, etc.).

It is not always detrimental to produce acid as it is part of our body's normal functioning. Acid only becomes a problem to our health when it builds up so much that there are no longer enough alkaline resources to deal with it. A lack of alkaline minerals and other substances plays a major role in creating a pH imbalance and if these substances are not replenished in some way, through foods especially, the resulting excess acidity can lead to poor health.

When we consider acid/alkaline (pH) balance, the most important area of the body is the blood. The pH of the blood must be kept within very narrow limits to prevent serious consequences to health. The body's homeostatic control mechanism, therefore, causes any excess acid found in the bloodstream to be immediately removed and deposited in the surrounding tissues in order to maintain the blood pH within its narrow limits. The pH environment of the surrounding tissues is not as critical, so the body's innate protective mechanism uses them as a storage place for the extra acid. Frequent off-loading of acid from the blood over a period of time can eventually lead to arthritis as the acid builds up, crystallizes and then attacks the joints, muscles and soft tissues.

This accumulation of acid in joints was made evident in a 2010 research study.[2] The pH level of joints was investigated and it was found that if a joint had a lower level of bicarbonate (an alkaline substance), this correlated with a significant increase in inflammation of the area. The research also discovered a link between the acidity of a joint and abnormalities that show up in blood tests, particularly when markers of inflammation such as C-Reactive Protein are found to be present.

Influences on acid/alkaline balance

There are many reasons why the body's pH may become imbalanced. These are the common ones that most people can identify with:

- diet
- digestive problems
- stress
- overuse of medications
- being overweight
- excessive exercise.

Diet

A typical Western diet includes a high level of processed foods and a lack of fresh, seasonal produce. Such a diet is deficient in essential fats, fibre and trace nutrients. When whole foods – in other words, foods which have undergone a minimum of processing – are lacking, the enzymes and fibre vital for digestion are also lacking, putting a strain on the digestive system. This, combined with a lack of vital vitamins and minerals, tilts the balance of the body towards excess acidity, which then leads to acid levels building up in the tissues, the joints, the muscles and so on.

Digestive problems

When you have any digestive problem, you may be unable to absorb nutrients from foods readily. Conditions such as irritable bowel syndrome, slow or fast transit time (the time taken for food to pass through the digestive tract and residues to be excreted), coeliac disease, eating the wrong foods at the wrong time, insufficient stomach acid, inadequate digestive enzymes, problems with the gut wall integrity (leaky gut syndrome), latent bacterial or fungal infections in the gut, poor balance of healthy bacteria – all these disorders lead to a decrease in the uptake of nutrients from food and quickly use up existing nutrients. The end result is that there is a deficiency of alkaline minerals, which again tilts the balance towards excess acidity.

Stress

More often than not, the onset of arthritis comes shortly after a very stressful time such as a bereavement, house move, relationship breakup, etc. Such an event is a common trigger for arthritis and plays a major role in worsening any existing symptoms. You will see in a moment how stress causes acid to be produced in the body and this is why your symptoms can feel a lot worse during or following a period of stress. To understand this, it helps to look at what is happening in the body when it is pushed to the limit. The nervous system is involved and it plays an important role in pH balance.

The nervous system is yet another example of the body's great protective mechanisms – it is critical to your survival. The nervous system is in 'sympathetic' mode when you are stressed; this is otherwise known as the 'fight or flight' state. The sympathetic nervous system is jolted into action in order to enable you to run away from threats or give you the strength to fight when you need it. The nervous system is in 'parasympathetic' mode when you are peaceful and calm; this is known as the 'rest and repair' state, and in this state your body can heal itself, repair any damage and recover its equilibrium from the day's challenges. It is crucially important to have balance between the two modes to avoid a situation of ill-health, not only from arthritis.

The sympathetic mode causes acid to be produced, while the parasympathetic mode has the opposite effect and is alkalizing to your body. These two modes or branches within your nervous system don't tend to work simultaneously – you are either predominantly in one state or the other. Relaxation, breathing exercises and calming activities such as yoga can bring you to a more 'parasympathetic' state, whereas ongoing stress, work, family issues, anxiety and worry can cause the 'sympathetic' state to dominate. In a sympathetic state, the body produces more acid than normal and puts extra strain on the alkaline reserves.

When the sympathetic nervous system is overactive, it exhausts the body. Its natural healing systems become impaired and the result can be chronic disease such as arthritis. A typical naturopathic programme for someone with arthritis might include nutrients to support their stressful lifestyle as a core component of their treatment. Removing the cause of stress is often recommended, but this can be very complex at times and may be impossible to achieve in the short term, whereas specific nutrients enable the body to cope better and be protected from the harmful effects of stress.

Typical work patterns and daily stresses deplete the body of nutrients such as B vitamins and magnesium; these are the very vitamins and minerals needed to help you cope with stress! B vitamins provide support for the nervous system and the adrenal glands – the glands responsible for how the body copes with stress. Magnesium is an alkaline mineral; it becomes depleted in the face of constant stress.

If an arthritic joint is treated in isolation, then as long as the underlying stress is still there, recovery is unlikely. Understanding the driving force behind joint problems is a big step to recovery as, once you have identified what that driving force is for you, you can begin to deal with it.

Overuse of medications

The overuse of medications often prescribed for digestive troubles, such as antacids and antibiotics, can interfere with the absorption of alkaline minerals and other nutrients. They can put stress on the liver, where detoxification from acidic wastes takes place; the liver becomes unable to perform its job efficiently. Use of such medication masks the initial symptoms, yet detrimental effects may still occur even though the problem seems to be solved.

Being overweight

Obese or overweight people are at an increased risk of osteoarthritis. The obvious reason why this can lead to arthritis is that being overweight means it simply becomes increasingly difficult to carry your own weight. Excess weight can be due to poor diet, lack of exercise or faulty metabolism, such as low thyroid function. Weight reduction can play an important role in recovery from arthritis.

The other – less obvious – reason why excess weight can be a problem is related to how fat acts in the body. Excess fat sets off processes in the body which promote inflammation, particularly in the area known as 'visceral abdominal fat' – the fat surrounding the organs in the middle of the body. The inflammation caused by excess fat draws on alkaline resources. The end result is to deplete the natural alkalizing capability of the whole body. More acid continues to build up, causing more inflammation, and the cycle continues.

Many toxins are stored within body fat, so reducing body fat should improve overall health and well-being while also reducing strain on the joints. It is important to follow responsible advice about weight loss and attempt a gradual, sustainable reduction rather than undergoing a drastic food limiting programme.

Of course, if arthritis has taken hold, our ability to exercise is limited, but gentle exercise of one kind or another is crucial to bringing the body back into pH balance.

Excessive exercise

Excessive exercise may in itself lead to an excess of lactic acid; we experience this as cramp. It is all about balance – if you don't exercise your joints frequently then poor circulation can result and degenerative changes will start to occur within the joint itself. However, if you overdo it or do not supply sufficient protective nutrients through sensible eating and a good supplement regime, then excessive exercise may lead to problems. Inappropriate exercise can also cause mechanical stress to the joints.

Reducing acidity

To enable recovery and prevent further damage to the joints, excess acidity from all its various sources must be reduced. Taking painkillers or anti-inflammatory drugs might help at this stage to mask the symptoms but over the longer term it is important to address the root cause of the problem, which is the acid. By addressing this, making changes to your diet and possibly your lifestyle, and taking specific nutritional food supplements to increase your alkaline resources, it is possible to regain optimal acid/alkaline balance throughout the body. As the excess acid becomes neutralized, symptoms disappear and, as an added bonus, your general health often becomes much improved.

An arthritic joint is usually not an isolated problem. It has often become damaged as a consequence of diet or lifestyle, or due to some trauma that has affected the metabolism of the whole body. It is crucial to view the affected joint as just a part of the whole bodily system; more joints may become susceptible to inflammation unless the whole body is encouraged into a more balanced acid/alkaline state. Viewing your body's health in its entirety is crucial to understanding how to successfully recover from arthritis and is a fundamental principle of natural medicine.

In the forthcoming chapters I will explain the various ways of addressing these underlying causes and help you to formulate your own recovery plan.

2

Natural treatment for arthritis: the three-category principle

As I have already said, I believe that the most effective way to achieve recovery from arthritis is to treat the body as a whole using naturopathic principles. In this chapter we will look at what exactly that entails, and I will explain the three-category principle of treatment for arthritis.

What is naturopathy?

The fundamental aim of naturopathy is to uncover the root cause of disease by viewing people as individuals, rather than just as collections of symptoms.

When trying to find the right treatment for an individual, the process considers not only a person's diet but also his or her lifestyle, hobbies, work and emotional, mental and physical health. When the person is treated as a whole, rather than just as a 'knee' or a 'hip', these factors are brought to the fore; the pieces of the puzzle come together to explain why that person is in the state that they are now in. The process of recovery carefully unpeels these layers of the disease and gets to the root of it, healing each layer and correcting the body's functions. The pain and inflammation will diminish and subside until they eventually clear totally and the person no longer suffers with arthritis.

One of the fundamental aspects of naturopathic treatment of arthritis is to restore the nutrient levels within the body. In most cases, this is not achieved through the diet alone, making it necessary to use dietary supplements. These may include vitamins, minerals, trace elements, proteins, herbs and plants.

How do natural supplements differ from pharmaceutical drugs?

There is a great deal of controversy today about the use of natural medicine and whether it is tested and assessed as comprehensively as pharmaceutical drugs are. Understanding the differences between the philosophies of natural and orthodox medicine may help to explain why this is the case.

Pharmaceutical drugs are rigorously tested and undergo an extensive programme to evaluate their action, usage and safety. This process results in a marketable drug that has undergone many clinical trials to ensure its suitability and safety in treating a particular disease or symptom.

It is not easy to do equivalent testing on natural products as there are so many additional factors involved. For example, there are many substances or compounds within plants and foods that give additional benefits when taking them. Some of these are known, and some remain unknown: how can we be sure we know absolutely everything about the way nature works? All products, natural or otherwise, are chosen for their active ingredient; however, the product in question may also contain some of these additional useful factors within the natural composition of the food or plant from which it originated.

To illustrate this concept, let us take a look at a supplement that is derived from pineapple. This fruit contains an enzyme called bromelain that is useful to us as both an anti-inflammatory and a digestive aid. The pineapple fruit also contains many other natural compounds that enhance the function of the active component, bromelain. These naturally occurring substances help bromelain to be absorbed and used efficiently within the body. You may find in good quality supplements that there is a proportion of bromelain, but that also on the ingredients list will be concentrated pineapple. The manufacturer has taken the extract (bromelain) but knows that it will be more effective if the whole pineapple concentrate is added, as it is within the whole pineapple that these other substances are present. When foods or plants are used as medicines, it is a principle of naturopathy to leave them in as natural a state as possible in order to gain the best possible outcome.

Pharmaceutical drugs are much more simplistic in that they act on a specific target in the body to produce a specific result or action.

Although simple for testing purposes, often little regard is given to the other effects, known as 'side effects', they may have in the body. Once a process in the body is interfered with in this way, there are bound to be consequences. For example, let's consider a commonly prescribed drug for arthritis, diclofenac.

Its action is: To decrease pain and inflammation in rheumatic disease and musculoskeletal disorders.

Its side effects are: gastrointestinal discomfort, nausea, diarrhoea, bleeding and ulceration, rash, bronchospasm, headaches, dizziness, nervousness, depression, drowsiness, insomnia, vertigo, hearing disturbances, fluid retention, raised blood pressure, kidney and liver problems (as listed in the *British National Formulary*[1]).

As it acts in the body on a specific pain mechanism, a medicine may also affect many different parts of the body. This is how side effects occur. Modern drugs like diclofenac can provide much-needed pain relief and reduce inflammation, but the benefits must be weighed up against the risks. Common sense tells us that long-term use is more likely to produce side effects and risks are likely to increase as time goes on. It is also a normal progression of treatment to increase the dose of the drug as it becomes harder to control the symptoms. With that in mind, I feel that the long-term solution for arthritis lies with restoring the body's normal functioning using natural means, rather than depending on strong medications.

Nutritional supplements are preparations intended to supplement your diet and provide nutrients such as vitamins, minerals, fibre, fatty acids or amino acids that may be missing or that you may not be consuming in sufficient quantities. As such, they usually correct a deficiency of that necessary substance, which then allows a biological event or process to return to normal functioning. Pharmaceutical drugs, on the other hand, introduce a 'foreign' chemical into the body that 'mimics' or replaces a certain natural substance.

The side effects of nutritional therapy are generally positive health outcomes, such as increased energy, normalizing of weight, better skin condition, etc. The negative effects felt throughout some stages of the treatment are due to the body detoxifying and offloading the acidic substances that are causing the condition. These are termed flare-ups, and you tend to feel a lot better after this process has taken place. I would not consider them to be a side effect but rather a process you must go through in order to get the disease out of your system. There is no such thing as a miracle cure (unfortunately!) and there is no suppression of symptoms involved in natural treatment; therefore you should expect to have some difficult spells as you are healing. If you support your body's own natural healing systems, however, ultimately your symptoms should not return. You will achieve a *sustainable* recovery.

You can use the information within this book to build your own supplement regime. Many people will achieve successful outcomes by following the recommendations given. If you don't feel you are progressing, read carefully the chapter at the end of this book on troubleshooting. The human body has an enormous capability to heal itself – you just need to give it what it needs.

Finally, a couple of words of caution:

- There may be some cases in which a nutritional supplement or herb is not suitable to take alongside your medication. I suggest if you are on a lot of medication or your situation is not straightforward that you consult our clinic or a nutritional therapist to help you. Most of the content of this book is suitable for use alongside typical prescriptions, but it is important to be aware of the possible interactions between the two forms of medicine.

- A word on safety. If your joint pain is undiagnosed, it is strongly recommended that you initially consult your GP. Never presume the source of your pain or self-diagnose, as this might lead you into a dangerous situation. It is essential to consult your doctor if you are having symptoms of excruciating pain, sudden-onset pain or any changes regarding your pain or mobility. Seeking a diagnosis from your doctor or consultant is important so that other illnesses can be ruled out. Useful tests such as blood tests and X-rays can be ordered; in some cases you may have to take a drug or a combination of drugs in order to stabilize acute symptoms before seeking a long-term solution.

Taking charge of your own health is vitally important to reclaiming your mobility, your sense of well-being and your ability to live your life the way you want.

The three-category principle of arthritis recovery

Successful natural treatment of arthritis, in my view, is based on combining various methods to produce the end result. In an ideal world, there would be one miracle product that would cure arthritis, but I do not believe this wish will ever materialize because true success relies on the incorporation of a multitude of factors into a comprehensive treatment. No single item can possibly affect all the underlying systems in arthritis to provide a worthwhile cure. Only temporary relief from symptoms can be attained using a single product, whether it is a drug or a supplement.

All natural products, remedies and solutions for arthritis can be classified into one of three categories:

1 nutrients that alkalize the body;
2 nutrients to repair the joint structures;
3 nutrients to relieve inflammation and pain.

Later on I will outline the various treatments that fit into each of these three categories. My philosophy is simple – take at least one element from each of the three categories and you will be on the right path to recovery. Miss out any of the categories and you may find relief, but you are unlikely to achieve a long-term cure.

I already take glucosamine – is this enough?

Glucosamine is one of the more popular supplements for joint pain. According to the above classification, this is a Category 2 nutrient as it helps to replenish the cartilage around the joint and also prevent further degeneration. You may feel some relief by taking glucosamine on a daily basis, only to find that if you stop taking it your symptoms return. Why is this? Well, quite simply, it's because factors from the other categories are not being included at the same time; therefore, it is very difficult, if not impossible, for your arthritis to just disappear. Glucosamine can be a very useful supplement but the main point is this: use it as part of a combination natural treatment, i.e. alongside nutrients from Categories 1 and 3. Having said this, a great many people might well be happy with keeping their arthritis 'at bay' by simply continuing to take their glucosamine supplement. But why stop there? If, with a few further actions, you could achieve total remission of your arthritis and stabilize your joints for the future, then why be satisfied with this halfway solution? I personally feel it is because we are led to believe that there is no cure for arthritis and it is just not possible to rid yourself of the condition completely. I disagree.

In the next three chapters I will explain in detail how the natural treatment for arthritis works – and by using these guidelines you will be better informed on how to achieve the best possible outcome. There are many 'wonder cures' for arthritis that give hope to those with the disease, but too often they end in disappointment. Why they work for some and not for others may have more to do with other things an individual does that have just not been acknowledged. All the components I'll talk about should independently improve not only your arthritis, but your general health and well-being too.

All three categories must be addressed to give yourself the best opportunity for full and total recovery from arthritis. It is the combination of factors with which you are most likely to succeed.

Is there are a cure for arthritis?

We constantly hear that there is no cure for arthritis; conventional treatment is focused on 'managing' the symptoms of the condition. I have met many people who would say their arthritis was not well-managed; they are suffering, with no one to turn to. While the word 'cure' can be misleading, I have seen many times the impressive effects of natural treatment in removing all signs of arthritis over a period of time. For example, people can be in debilitating pain, unable to work and socialize, yet – with guidance – they achieve so much through natural treatment that they return to their previous healthy state with no remaining symptoms. At the end of this book I have included some case studies so you can read about some of our clinic patients and their recoveries. Of course, this is anecdotal. The medical establishment might argue that this is hearsay rather than a clinically evidenced way of overcoming arthritis. So I have also drawn together much of the latest scientific research, to build up that much-needed evidence.

No single supplement, drug or action provides a cure for arthritis even though these elements will have some effects on reducing the symptoms. A multitude of efforts should be undertaken to bring about complete and lasting remission.

3

Category 1:
alkalizing the body

I explained in Chapter 1 how excess acidity builds up in the body and starts to degrade joints, causing inflammation and pain. Category 1 remedies provide measures to combat excess acidity. There are many different acids and alkalis present in everyday food and drink, so what you consume can either have an acidic or an alkaline effect.

Alkali can neutralize or destroy acid, because alkali is chemically opposite to acid and cancels it out – therefore, it is extremely important to increase your intake of alkaline foods and drinks, and stop as far as possible your intake of acidic foods and drinks. Water can dilute acid in the body, rendering it less harmful – therefore, it makes sense to increase your intake of water.

These are vital dietary changes, but there are also a range of traditional naturopathic techniques to neutralize excess acid. These include taking cider vinegar drinks and Epsom salt baths.

Using dietary means to alkalize the body

Although this book focuses on the supplements available for arthritis, we cannot avoid referring to diet as this should form a crucial part of the treatment programme. Supplements are exactly that; supplements to the daily diet, not replacements for it. Therefore, the advice given in this book is only effective when implemented alongside a healthy diet. It is very important that I advise you on what a 'healthy' diet consists of, as this in itself is often misinterpreted.

In 2004, the Nutrition Society looked into the effects of diet on rheumatoid arthritis and 'it was demonstrated that lower intakes of fruit and vegetables and dietary vitamin C are associated with an increased risk of developing inflammatory polyarthritis'.[1] Many scientific reports agree that diet has a significant impact on arthritis, but the subject has been talked about for many years with great differences of opinion being expressed. Some people find that diet has a remarkable effect on their symptoms, while others struggle to notice any difference. I believe that everything you take into your body has an effect, positive or negative, on your well-being.

Consider that each and every time you consume something, it is an opportunity to provide your body with the materials it needs to heal itself. That is, after all, what we are trying to achieve with everything mentioned in this book: to provide your body with nutrients from foods, drinks and supplements that will enable it to do exactly what it is designed to do: heal itself.

The word diet often instils a great sense of dread. We imagine punishing restrictions and are often reluctant to try yet another wonder diet just in case we might experience the health benefits it claims to provide. Yes, diet is significant in a recovery programme; however, it doesn't need to be excessively restrictive, uninteresting and difficult to implement. This section largely provides information about what you *can* eat, rather than focusing too much on what to avoid. Try to see the dietary advice you will find here as an opportunity to venture into new realms of eating, choosing new foods, and simply enjoying your diet as it provides great benefits, not only to painful joints, but to the whole body.

There are restrictions to the diet, of course, as it involves eliminating particularly acidic foods. However, these restrictions are sensible; they do not include entire food groups and do not impose harsh calorific restrictions, as might be seen with other diets. I understand that dietary changes can be daunting and hard to stick to. If you find the advice particularly difficult to follow, one way of doing so is to observe an 80/20 rule: 80 per cent of your diet should be beneficial alkaline foods, leaving 20 per cent for the occasions when you want to eat something that is on the restricted, acidic list. More tips on how to make the diet work for you will follow later. Once you start seeing the results from the programme you should have more confidence in making changes.

This way of eating is suitable for all the family and should enhance your well-being whether you have arthritis or not. It is suitable for following on a long-term basis, and will not cause any nutrient deficiencies if done correctly. If you are overweight this type of diet should help reduce your weight – by normalizing the acid/alkaline balance of the body, it in turn encourages a healthy metabolism and functioning. By the same token, if you are underweight you should find you start to gain weight by choosing foods that encourage healthy functioning and healthy metabolism in the body.

As previously discussed, over-acidity is a major cause of arthritic joints. Excess acid accumulates in the body due to a variety of factors but long-term food habits play a major role. This is why a dietary approach to arthritis can be so successful: it addresses the acid/alkaline imbalance and in so doing addresses one of the major causes of arthritis. Tackling the underlying cause or combination of causes is the way to long-term, sustainable recovery as the factors driving your arthritis disappear.

The following recommendations are based on knowledge of the foods themselves and on the clinical effects I have observed in practice. The beginning is the most difficult stage, but once you start to reap the benefits it becomes so much easier and more enjoyable.

Beneficial foods

The following foods can all be eaten freely and should be incorporated into your new healthy diet. Individual benefits are mentioned as many of these foods have great qualities; they should almost be seen as medicine. As the father of medicine, Hippocrates, famously believed, 'Thy food is thy medicine and thy medicine is thy food'. This ancient principle is equally valid in today's world as increasing numbers of people develop diseases and ailments that may be induced by their diet and lifestyle.

Grains and cereals

Whole grains, as unprocessed as possible, will tend to increase the alkalinity of the body. Natural, whole grains, like other whole foods, contain the minerals needed to buffer any acidic portions of the food. If the grain is stripped away, these alkaline minerals are removed, and as a result the grain has more of an acidic effect on the body. Unprocessed grains are far more beneficial for the digestion, providing roughage to prevent constipation and other difficulties. They are rich in B vitamins; whole grains are a far better source of this beneficial vitamin group than processed grains. Look for 'whole' wheat when you buy pasta and bread, 'whole' oats, 'wholegrain' barley, 'wholegrain' rye.

Varying the type of grain or cereals consumed will not only provide a far broader selection of nutrients but will prevent the over-consumption of any one type, e.g. wheat, which can in itself put extra strain on the body. The following are all beneficial grains:

Wild rice For its very potent alkalizing benefits and richness in naturally occurring trace minerals.

Quinoa For its relatively high protein content. Quinoa is very light and easy to digest. It is rather bland tasting so it is advisable to use herbs to season it and have it as an accompaniment to stronger, full flavoured foods. Cook in a similar way to rice.

Spelt An ancient variety of the wheat grain. Some wheat intolerant people get on very well with this grain. If using spelt flour, use as plain wheat flour.

Buckwheat This does not contain gluten and is actually a seed rather than a grain. Buckwheat makes lovely pancakes that taste like traditional French crêpes. Use it for a breakfast variation, instead of wheat.

Oats These have many benefits. Oats have become a superfood in themselves, with more and more research focusing on their health applications. Oats are now known to benefit high cholesterol, digestive disorders and skin problems among many more, and new findings are being revealed all the time. Oats contain mucilage, a gooey substance that helps to cleanse the digestive tract and bind toxic residues, improving the overall health of the bowel. This may be of particular importance to people with rheumatoid arthritis, as they often have some level of imbalance within their digestive tract. A good bowl of porridge from 'whole' oats is a great way to start the day.

Millet Porridge can be made with millet flakes. This grain is suitable for gluten-free diets. The uses of millet are similar to those of oats.

Sprouted grains and seeds These are available 'ready to eat' in some supermarkets and health food shops. The sprouted version of a grain, bean or seed is consumed once it has been soaked and fermented. In a process that imitates nature, the grain is constantly soaked and then dried in a warm environment until it sprouts; by the time sprouting takes place, all the anti-nutrients that cause digestive problems – such as phytates, tannins, complex sugars, gluten and related proteins – have been partially broken down into simple components that are more readily digested. 'Sprouted grain' bread can usually be tolerated by people who normally cannot eat wheat. Mung bean sprouts, alfalfa sprouts, mixed sprouts and chickpea sprouts are all excellent sprouted seeds. Sprouted grains are a very rich nutrient source. As they are so small, many can be consumed at one mealtime, thereby increasing the nutrient intake further; some say their nutritional value is as much as 20 to 30 times better than that of the mature grain. Add to stir fries or salads.

Fish

Fish provides an excellent source of protein, which as you will see later is essential for the repair of damaged joints. Some types of fish also offer anti-inflammatory benefits, particularly the oily fish, rich in the essential fat omega 3. Oily fish include sardines, mackerel, wild salmon, herring and anchovies (although anchovies can be salty).

White fish, such as cod, haddock, trout and bass, are not an especially abundant source of omega 3 but are a useful source of dietary protein. White fish are normally easy on the digestive system and may be particularly useful if your appetite is affected by constant pain.

Canned fish such as sardines, pilchards and salmon are very good as you eat the bones too, and they are a good source of natural calcium.

Have fish steamed, baked or grilled, rather than fried. Do not have deep-fried fish.

Shellfish, such as prawns, mussels, langoustine or crab, are good sources of omega 3 fatty acids as well as minerals such as zinc, iodine, selenium and copper.

Don't eat only one variety of fish or shellfish regularly and do not eat raw fish. Due to pollution in the seas and oceans around the world, heavy metals and other pollutants are now prevalent to a greater or lesser extent in all types of fish. Vary the type of fish you eat to minimize the possible effect of such contaminants on your body.

Poultry

Free range chicken and turkey are excellent sources of protein which also provide a modest level of anti-inflammatory nutrients, particularly within the darker leg meats. A lower standard than free range is not advisable as such poultry tends to be intensively farmed with the use of antibiotics, growth hormones and certain additives. These methods are not conducive to human health. I recommend you eat only good quality poultry. If price is an issue for you it is preferable to occasionally eat organic, free-range chicken or turkey rather than eating poorer quality meat more often.

Vegetables

With the exception of tomatoes, all vegetables can be eaten in abundance. Steaming vegetables will retain far more nutrients than boiling them, so this is a good option. Quick stir-frying is also suitable as it leaves the vegetables quite crisp with their nutrients intact. Green leafy vegetables such as broccoli, cabbage and kale should be eaten regularly, as these have a gentle hormone balancing activity in addition to their antioxidant value. (I will talk about antioxidants later on.) Try to vary the vegetables you eat each week but have at least three to five portions daily if possible. Fresh-frozen vegetables are a fine alternative if you live alone and have difficulty getting to the shops. Supermarkets often sell frozen organic vegetables and their nutrients are fairly well preserved if freshly frozen.

One way of varying the intake of vegetables within your diet is to purchase a weekly box that is delivered to the door. This can be a cost-effective way of buying vegetables in season and the quality tends to be very good.

Fruits

Choose from apples, bananas, melons, apricots, peaches and avocados. Have one serving each day. If you eat dried fruits, such as apricots, it is best to limit the amount to just a few, as the concentrated sugars within the dried fruit may add to the acidity of your body.

Desserts

Yes, the reduced-acid diet includes a dessert section! We all have times when a little indulgence is necessary, and if you know how to make your favourite desserts healthier or are simply able to find alternatives to finish a meal off, you will be able to continue enjoying this luxury.

Cream, milk, sugar, excess wheat and butter should be avoided, but here are some good substitutes for common dessert ingredients such as these:

- *Cream* – soya cream, oat cream, natural live yoghurt, tofu cream/ silken tofu
- *Milk* – almond milk, hazelnut milk, oat milk, rice milk or soya milk, skimmed cow's milk

- *Sugar* – xylitol, agave, blackstrap organic molasses, barley malt extract, rice syrup, apple juice, honey or dark sugars as unprocessed as possible
- *Breadcrumbs* – ground almonds (or other nuts), wheatgerm, oatbran, ground flaxseed/linseed
- *Flour* – spelt flour, gluten-free flour, ground nuts (almonds work well), oatbran, wheatgerm
- *Butter* – coconut oil can make a delicious alternative to butter in baking.

It may take a bit of creativity but you can still eat desserts occasionally without impeding your progress.

Drinks

The importance of drinking sufficient fluids cannot be stressed too much, but what is the right fluid to drink? Our bodies consist of around 55 to 70 per cent water and without it we would cease to exist, so water is very important. One can go without food for many days and weeks – even longer in some cases – but one cannot survive more than a couple of days without water.

We know that if we do not drink adequate fluids, the residues of digestion and metabolism build up in the body and we cannot clear the toxins away, i.e. we become constipated – the bowel does not perform its natural function of removing wastes. The body's natural way of minimizing the effect of waste products is to dilute them in water, and water is used to transport such wastes through the body and to the outside.

When you have arthritis, toxins impair the way your body's cells are able to interact with water and water retention is often a problem. Let's think about this a little more carefully. Water is the carrier of minerals in the body, and proper mineral balance is vital to normal health. So it is helpful to add minerals to the water that you drink. Your body's cells are then more able to interact with mineral-enriched water and, consequently, hydration is achieved more easily. So how do you enrich your drinking water easily with minerals?

- *Diluted cider vinegar drinks* These rehydrate the body. Drink three glasses daily if you have arthritis or one daily for general well-being. Add one teaspoon of honey to each glass unless you are diabetic.
- *Trace mineral supplements* Available from health food stores, these liquid supplements – sourced usually from mineral-rich lakes or waters – deliver a natural spectrum of trace minerals.

Other beneficial drinks include the following:

- *Herbal teas* e.g. chamomile, peppermint, fennel. These calming teas aid digestion and settle the nervous system before sleep.
- *Green tea* This can be very powerful for reducing arthritic symptoms and the latest research reflects this attribute: a study published in the *Journal of Nutrition* found that green tea possessed anti-inflammatory properties and caused changes in arthritis-related immune responses, suggesting its potential for the treatment of rheumatoid arthritis and possibly other types of autoimmune arthritis.[2]
- *Ginger tea* Simply grate some fresh root ginger into hot water and drink after meals. It aids digestion and is known to have an anti-inflammatory effect.
- *Apple tea* Steep apple peelings in boiling water for five to seven minutes.
- *Almond milk* I recommend this as a tasty alternative to cow's milk. The drink can be sweetened using a little honey, molasses or agave syrup.
- *White tea* Similar to green tea but lower in caffeine, this type of tea is rich in antioxidants to help fight inflammation.
- *Nettle tea* With its high mineral content and mild diuretic action, nettle is one of nature's few kidney tonics. It is alkalizing to the body.
- *Dandelion tea* This plant is known to support liver and kidney function and may be useful in draining excess fluid from the body. It is potential very useful for those with fluid retention, high blood pressure and joint swelling.

Foods that should be avoided

Eliminate foods that produce an acidic effect in the body. These include:

- × citrus fruits;
- × beef and all beef products, such as corned beef, beefburgers, pastrami, beef stock cubes, oxtail, calf's liver, etc.;
- × pork and all pork products, including sausages, bacon, ham, gammon, prosciutto, pancetta, pâté, terrine, chorizo, salami, spare ribs, etc.;
- × tomatoes – all varieties, including sauces, ketchup, tinned, purée, etc., whether raw or cooked as in pizza;
- × cheese (with the exception of skimmed milk cheese products such as cottage cheese);
- × refined carbohydrates – these are the 'whites': white flour, white pasta

(e.g. spaghetti and lasagne), white rice, white bread, white sugar;

x processed foods – ready meals, boxed meals, packaged cakes and biscuits, crisps, frozen dinners, sweets, crackers, frozen chips, fish sticks, pies and pastries;

x hydrogenated fats and trans fats or trans-fatty acids – e.g. those found in margarines, fried foods, takeaways, fast foods;

x excessive sugar intake – in hot drinks, cakes, biscuits, processed foods, tinned foods, pre-made sauces, etc.;

x cakes and biscuits made with white flour, white sugar, etc.;

x chocolate – milk, plain, white and dark;

x excessive wheat. Wheat is the basis of most pastas and breads and is an ingredient of many prepared sauces and gravies. It is easy to have too much wheat in your diet and this may have negative effects. Incorporate grains other than wheat into your diet;

x dairy foods. Switch to skimmed milk or try an alternative such as almond milk, soya milk or rice milk;

x alcohol, including all wine, spirits, lager and beer. Avoid alcohol in cooking too;

x coffee;

x tea (black);

x soft drinks and 'diet' drinks;

x fizzy or carbonated drinks;

x any food or drink containing artificial sweeteners such as aspartame, acesulfame K, NutraSweet, Neotame, Splenda, etc. Artificial sweeteners can be particularly harmful. These are often hidden in cordials, sugar-free options of all foods, cereals, etc.;

x additives. Generally speaking, artificial additives to foods will likely increase acid accumulation in the body. These include those used to preserve food for longer, enhance the flavours, add colour, etc. If you see many items you don't recognize on the label, then my advice would be to disregard the product and find a more natural option;

x fruit juices and dried fruits. When fruits are juiced, the resulting juice has a high level of natural sugars. This sugar then produces acid. The same applies to dried fruits – the natural fruit sugars within have been concentrated so that your intake of sugar is far higher than when you have the un-dried version of the fruit. Aside from this issue, additives such as sulphur dioxide are often added to retain the natural colour of the fruit and prevent browning. This is particularly common in dried apricots, to retain their orange colour. Organic dried apricots are, in fact, naturally brown when you purchase them – they do not contain this additive.

The 'grey areas' of the alkaline diet

In addition to the above list, some other foods need to be considered. It has often been suggested over the years that foods within the nightshade family – potatoes, tomatoes, aubergines and peppers – have a detrimental effect on people with arthritis. As mentioned above, tomatoes are very acid and should be avoided. However, in my experience, potatoes, aubergines and peppers do not have a negative effect, although some people may have an intolerance to them in the same way that some people cannot eat onions or garlic.

Meat

Generally speaking, all meats tend to be acid-forming in the body. However, meat provides valuable benefits – it is a very useful source of high-quality protein that provides a complete range of essential amino acids, necessary for healthy functioning of the body.

Pork and beef are on the acid list and should therefore be avoided, along with all the associated products containing elements of either meat, such as ham, sausages, bacon, pork pies, beef burgers, etc. Lamb is a younger animal when slaughtered for its meat when compared with sheep, pigs or cows. Its meat tends to be less acid-forming and so can be eaten occasionally as the red meat option.

Fruit

It is generally agreed that citrus fruits are acid-forming, although lemons are often reported to be alkaline; however, this may well be only when they are taken in isolation such as within a fasting regime. When mixed with any other food I believe lemons have an acidic effect in the body. Foods such as pineapples and papaya contain beneficial enzymes (the action of enzymes is explained in Chapter 5) that have an anti-inflammatory action in the body, so for some people they may be very useful. However, others are unable to tolerate these fruits so well. Berries, particularly the darker coloured varieties, are rich in antioxidants – substances very beneficial for people with arthritis. However, some berries may be acid-forming in the body and, therefore, are not beneficial if you are trying to overcome arthritis. The fact is that natural foods are not simple compounds that only have one effect. Whether a particular food is harmful to you depends very much on your general metabolism, digestion and state of health.

I would advise you to err on the side of caution and steer clear of the foods in this 'grey area'. It would be a shame to routinely include them in your diet only to find that your arthritis does not improve. You would never know if it might be because of these foods, so my advice is to leave them alone until your symptoms have cleared.

How to implement the diet

At first, make changes slowly. Aim each week to try something new and eliminate a few more acid-forming foods.

If your mobility is very impaired and you find it difficult standing to cook for any length of time, enlist the help of someone who can prepare big batches of meals that can be stored in the freezer. A family member or a friend would be ideal, even if only once a fortnight to restock your freezer for you. Each day, a meal can be reheated in the oven with minimal effort, allowing you to follow the diet. If this is not easy for you because you live in a remote area or don't have such support available, then perhaps focus on raw foods that need little preparation.

Know that there will always be something you find difficult to remove from your diet. The most common stumbling block, in my experience, is tomatoes, as there is no obvious replacement for them and they are abundantly used in many cooking sauces, salads and other recipes. They also happen to be extremely acid-forming, so it is essential to eliminate them from your diet until you have recovered. Do your best to adhere to the diet. The road to recovery is not necessarily easy; try to remain focused on the positive aspects of your new eating regime and the effects it will have.

Many people with arthritis also have intolerances to certain foods. These people might be reluctant to change their dietary routine as whenever they have done so before, it has always upset their system and caused undesirable effects. Such effects might include skin troubles, stomach and bowel upsets, headaches, lack of energy, and more. This reluctance is understandable but, if you feel like this, take a food intolerance test to identify the specific foods that your system cannot tolerate at the moment. For details, see Useful addresses at the end of this book.

Think realistically what you can achieve. Even small changes can make a great impact on your arthritis. Use these changes to help motivate you to take the diet to the next level and become even stricter. It can be very satisfying to have such control over your own symptoms by adjusting your diet.

Read labels. Often foods contain ingredients you might not expect. Try to get in the habit of looking at labels as this will help you make the right choice. The offending ingredients are often not even necessary and it can be very simple to find the same product without them.

Review your diet every couple of months and see what you can do better; try to always aim higher and not get stuck eating a bland diet each day with little variation.

Aim for an 80/20 alkalizing diet. Try eating according to the principles of the reduced-acid diet for a minimum of 80 per cent of the time, allowing yourself up to 20 per cent of the time to eat whatever is presented to you. This will allow you to socialize with friends or family without feeling too much of a burden. Provided your daily routine is to stick to a reduced-acid diet, what happens when you are on holiday or out of your normal environment should have little effect.

If you do happen to eat something too acidic, take an extra glass of cider vinegar before the day is over. This should help to counteract it so your progress won't be set back. The stricter you are, the better your chances of a speedier recovery.

The acid/alkaline diet is complex. It is not possible to draw a line so that all foods and drinks fall into either the acid or alkaline section – or at least there would be much debate. You only have to look at the internet to find lists of acid foods, none of which will be consistent and in agreement. Acidity is more of a sliding scale than it is a single description. Predominantly acid foods also contain alkaline components and the reverse is also true. It isn't possible to avoid all acid foods, but what is achievable is to rebalance your diet so that it leans more in an alkaline than an acidic direction.

Taking a positive approach to diet will help a great deal with the adjustments. The next section details traditional methods of alkalizing the body.

Cider vinegar

Cider vinegar is an ancient folk remedy with many associated health claims. In Ancient Greece in 400 BC, Hippocrates, 'the father of medicine', prescribed apple cider vinegar mixed with honey as a health tonic, an antibiotic and an energizing elixir. It has been used by many others in the naturopathic field since then.

Apple cider vinegar is an embodiment of the popular saying, 'An apple a day keeps the doctor away'. This vinegar not only contains all the concentrated goodness of the apples from which it was made, but also the enzymes and beneficial acids produced by the fermentation process that turns the juice of the apple into vinegar. Cider vinegar is a fairly well-known remedy with much anecdotally reported success in relieving the aches and pains associated with arthritis.

Cider vinegar provides minerals to the body in an easily absorbed form, and these minerals then counteract the excess acidity. This nourishing drink is reputed to dissolve the acid crystals that lodge painfully within the joints of someone with arthritis and, by putting these acids into solution, enables the body to excrete them.

Let's consider the extra benefits cider vinegar offers; this will show how appropriate it is to incorporate into your daily routine. Often arthritis goes hand in hand with digestive troubles. Cider vinegar is particularly beneficial for the digestive system as it helps to normalize the level of stomach acid, enabling the effective breakdown of foods. Because it is rich in enzymes, cider vinegar further aids the digestion of foods as, once the food gets past the stomach, enzymes are needed. Many people produce insufficient enzymes from their pancreas and have symptoms such as indigestion, wind and abdominal pain. Daily cider vinegar consumption should benefit such people.

Cider vinegar provides potassium, one of the alkalizing minerals. A report for doctors known as the *Townsend Letter* once mentioned a research study determining that whole-body potassium levels are significantly lower in older people with arthritis.[3] The study found that in some, the levels of potassium were only about half of what is considered to be normal, indicating that their bodies were in an excessively acidic state. Considering its cellular function within the body, potassium is one of the most important neutralizers of acidity: it is drawn out of cells to neutralize the acidity of the surrounding tissues. When this process is overburdened, due to persistent excess acid, the potassium levels become far too low to be drawn back into cells. It is very unlikely that the people studied in this research were deficient in potassium because of their diets, as potassium is present in many foods. It is much more likely that their body's constant fight against acidity used up potassium so quickly that it became depleted. Perhaps the normalization of potassium levels in the body is one reason why cider vinegar seems to work so well as a remedy for arthritis.

Isn't cider vinegar acid?

A frequent misconception is that, as all vinegars are acidic, cider vinegar causes your body to become excessively acidic. In fact the opposite is true. On the bottle, it is marked at around 5 per cent acidity, which often puts people off taking it as they wrongly believe that it will make their body too acid. However, the chemistry of what happens to the foods we eat is more complex. Whereas some foods and drinks remain acid and some alkaline, others actually switch from one to the other dependent on food combinations, i.e. what else is eaten within the same meal. Cider vinegar is one of the exceptions to the rule. It begins with 5 per cent acidity but it leaves a residual alkaline effect in the body. It is the only type of vinegar that behaves in this way; all other vinegars remain acid in the body and should not be used at all if you have arthritic joints. You should replace all other vinegars with cider vinegar when it is called for in cooking.

Cider vinegar is commonly drunk in combination with honey to increase its nutrient value. Honey contains minerals and enzymes as well as trace amounts of amino acids – all nutrients that benefit health. Honey is a natural antibiotic and is very useful in treating infections, both internally and topically, in other words on the skin.

The daily consumption of well-diluted cider vinegar and honey fits in well with the principles of eating unprocessed whole foods, using the nutritional benefits that nature provides us with.

Choosing a cider vinegar

When choosing cider vinegar, there are some important things to look out for:

- Ideally, find a cloudy product with some sediment. This is the best type to take, as what is known as the 'mother' – the visible dense strands within the liquid – contains extra nutrients. Some people make the mistake of filtering this out before drinking, but it holds

such great benefits that you should never remove it. If some sediment is left in your bottle at the end, always pour this into the next bottle.
- Look at the label for 'unpasteurized and unfiltered' cider vinegar.
- Organic brands are better as they have been produced from organic apples, without the use of any harmful chemicals in the production process. However, you may be lucky and find a small local producer who can supply you with his cider vinegar. If he is only a small producer he may not have an official organic certification, but ask if he uses chemicals, pesticides, etc., at any stage of production.
- Most supermarkets stock cider vinegar within the oils and vinegars section, although these may not contain 'mother'.
- Health food stores are a good source of cider vinegar in varying bottle sizes and brands.
- Do not use the tablet or capsule form of cider vinegar. This is widely available but will not have the same beneficial effects as drinking the diluted liquid. In order for the cider vinegar to perform its action of dissolving acid crystals from within affected joints, it has to be in solution. The tablets will not help in this way.

Dose

- For arthritis: 2 teaspoons (10 ml) well diluted in approximately 300ml water; 3 glasses daily, ideally 15 to 20 minutes before meals.
- For general health maintenance: use the same dilution as for arthritis but 1 glass daily should suffice.
- Add honey – dissolve 1 small teaspoon (5 ml) with hot water, then top up the glass with cold water before adding the cider vinegar.

Additional guidelines

- *Do not use boiling water* – heat may destroy some of the beneficial enzymes within the cider vinegar.
- *Diabetes* – if you cannot tolerate honey then please leave this out and have well-diluted cider vinegar alone.
- *Overweight* – you can double the amount of cider vinegar in each glass, i.e. 3 glasses daily with 4 teaspoons of cider vinegar in each.
- *Acidic conditions of the upper digestive tract, i.e. reflux/indigestion etc.* – start slowly, using only 1 teaspoon cider vinegar in 300 ml water at least. Sip slowly and gradually increase to the full dose and dilution over a couple of weeks.
- If taking water tablets, or if you have a stomach ulcer or hiatus hernia,

only 2 teaspoons (10 ml) cider vinegar should be taken in each drink.

- *Tooth enamel* – many people are concerned about the effect of cider vinegar on dental health, as the advice has always been that acidic drinks such as orange juice have a destructive effect on tooth enamel. In fact, as cider vinegar plays an important role in alkalizing the body, it has an overall beneficial effect, particularly on the acidity level of the gums which provide the groundwork for healthy teeth. If you have very poor dental health then you may drink the cider vinegar through a straw, although this may not be necessary.

Epsom salts (magnesium sulphate)

Bathing in Epsom salts has two distinct benefits. First, the baths provide a good dose of an alkalizing mineral, magnesium, which is absorbed readily via the skin. Second, they also provide the mineral sulphur, which is of great importance to the joints.

Epsom salts are a traditional remedy for a range of ailments. The absorption of magnesium keeps the body in an alkaline state and this is the main reason why they are so effective as a treatment for arthritis – the baths reduce the build-up of excess acidity. In addition, despite the simplicity of Epsom salt baths, each and every aspect holds its own advantages:

Water provides the ideal medium for effectively transporting sulphur and magnesium into the body, via the skin.

Heat provides muscle relaxation while opening the skin's pores to allow in the salt nutrients and drawing the toxins out. Heat also improves circulation.

Time Just 10 to 15 minutes three times each week allows you the personal space needed to focus on your active participation in your recovery. Stress will be handled more easily if the bath is taken in peace and quiet.

Underwater exercise It is far easier to mobilize a stiff joint using water for support than it is to perform any other exercise. Turn your ankles and wrists, lengthen and stretch your legs, feet and arms, roll your shoulders, hunch forwards and back to mobilize your spine, clench and stretch your fingers and toes. It is an active quarter of an hour!

Aside from these benefits, which any type of bath would provide, the medicinal quality of Epsom salts is due to the high content of the minerals, magnesium and sulphur.

Magnesium

In the treatment of arthritis, the primary role of magnesium is to alkalize the body tissues and joints. It has many further benefits:

- It helps those with osteoporosis or osteopenia (thinning of the bones), as it assists the uptake of calcium into the bone itself.
- It is a very effective muscle relaxant and can ease the tension caused by poor mobility and pain.
- Insomnia is a problem that can impair the body's ability to heal itself. Magnesium often restores a productive sleeping pattern and one tends to feels more refreshed and energetic on rising the following day.
- It is crucial for energy production in the body. A deficiency of magnesium can cause feelings of tiredness and lethargy.
- It is a very important mineral to nourish your nervous system and keep you calm. It is often named the 'anti-stress' mineral.
- It provides benefits to the cardiovascular system and may help to lower blood pressure and prevent hardening of the arteries.
- It is important in ensuring a healthy blood sugar level and may aid those with diabetes or hypoglycaemia.

Deficiencies of this important mineral are common. One way of assessing your magnesium level is the tongue test. Stick your tongue out and look in the mirror, trying to hold it still. If it shakes or trembles or ripples across the top then this may indicate a deficiency of magnesium. If you can successfully hold it still, then you are probably fine. Please note: this is not an accurate diagnostic method. Use it as a guide only.

Symptoms that may indicate a deficiency include the following:

- restless legs
- palpitations
- high blood pressure
- fatigue
- headaches
- migraines
- premenstrual symptoms
- osteoporosis or osteopenia

- blood sugar irregularities, i.e. becoming shaky or irritable when you are hungry
- sugar cravings.

People under stress are at particular risk as this situation causes the loss of magnesium from your body. For those with arthritis, magnesium is essential to buffer the excess acidity and support your nervous system while enabling good sleep and relaxation throughout your recovery period.

Sulphur

Many scientific studies indicate that sulphur is a vital joint nutrient and painkiller. Sulphur is important within the joint itself, being the fundamental building block of components of the joint such as cartilage. Bathing in Epsom salts provides the body with a useful form of sulphur which can be used by the body to normalize this process. The baths can be safely taken alongside painkillers, anti-inflammatory medications or steroids.

There is a substantial body of research backing up the usefulness of sulphur. A study in the Netherlands highlighted the importance of sulphur in the production of the joint cartilage components that often degrade in arthritis.[4] Just a small reduction in the sulphur concentration causes a significant reduction in the synthesis of these crucial cushioning joint substances, causing the eventual breakdown of the function of the joint. In 2010, another study observed a significant reduction of inflammation and cartilage breakdown when people with arthritis underwent sulphur-based spa therapies.[5] Joints affected by osteoarthritis tend to have a lower amount of sulphur within them.[6] Supplementing with sulphur over a three-month period significantly reduced the pain in those with osteoarthritis.[7]

Directions for Epsom salts baths

Bathe three times weekly. Prepare a hot bath and dissolve in it 400 g of Epsom salts. Bathe for 15 minutes, exercising all of your joints under the water. Do this in the evening, before bed, pat your skin dry, then keep warm and shower on rising the next day.

It is important not to rinse the body for at least 6 to 8 hours after a bath to ensure maximum absorption of the salts. After a bedtime bath, showering the following morning is essential to remove any acidic substances that may have been drawn to the skin's surface.

Cautions

Some people who take Epsom salts baths may experience sweating over-night. This is normal and is probably due to the detoxification induced by the bath. Reduce your baths to once weekly if it becomes problematic. This effect should diminish after time.

Many people with arthritis cannot get in or out of the bath, making this therapy difficult. An alternative is to take hand and foot baths in the solution, using 1 teacupful per bowl. This can be done up to four times daily.

The baths may not be suitable for people with cardiovascular health problems due to the heat of the bath. In such cases, reduce the temperature of the water.

Supplement alternatives

If for any reason you are unable to take Epsom salts baths, there are a number of other ways of getting the magnesium and sulphur you need:

Magnesium oral supplements   These are best taken at night, before bed. They are available in capsules, tablets or as homeopathic tissue salts for those who have trouble swallowing. When you are on holiday, or away from home, this is an easy alternative to bathing. Dosage: 200–600 mg daily of elemental magnesium.

Magnesium spray   This can be applied topically to the area of pain or stiffness, or alternatively can be sprayed anywhere on the body to provide a dose of magnesium via the skin. Products vary but generally speaking, it is best to use about 10 to 15 sprays twice daily to obtain a therapeutic benefit. You may find your skin tingles when the spray is first applied.

MSM (Methylsulphonylmethane)   A preparation that provides sulphur. It is available in capsules, powder or as a cream or gel for topical application directly to the joints or muscles affected.

Blackstrap molasses

Molasses is the nutrient-dense product of the sugar cane plant, once the sugar has been extracted. The process of extraction involves the crystallization and subsequent removal of the sugar, leaving behind the extremely nutritious residue that is known as molasses. Blackstrap molasses has undergone this crystallization process a number of times to ensure most traces of sugar are removed. Other types of molasses tend to contain more sugar, which is detrimental to arthritis, whereas blackstrap has a very low sugar content.

A natural sugar cane plant is extremely rich in nutrients due to its extremely long roots. These roots dig deep beneath the topsoil into the rich underlayers of the earth where they absorb substantial amounts of vitamins and minerals. The sugar that is extracted, which eventually becomes our table sugar, is significantly lacking in these nutrients. Darker sugars have undergone less processing and therefore retain some nutrients, but the only way to acquire the deep soil nutrients mentioned is by consuming molasses – what some would consider the waste product of sugar manufacture.

If molasses is incorporated into treatment for arthritis, it must be organic and it must be blackstrap. Other versions will not be suitable. Non-organic versions may have sulphites added during the manufacturing process, in which case they will not be suitable for daily intake.

Blackstrap molasses is a whole food source of many vitamins and minerals. It is a good source of calcium, iron, potassium and B vitamins, all of which are commonly deficient in those with arthritis. It also provides many other useful nutrients including copper, magnesium, chromium, manganese, molybdenum, zinc, phosphorus and vitamin E.

Many people with arthritis also have anaemia – lowered amounts of red blood cells. Molasses provides not only the iron to correct this but also B vitamins to assist the building of red blood cells.

Molasses aids the digestive system, which is often affected in those with arthritis. As the gut function impacts on the entire health of the body, including the joints, this benefit alone should indicate its use as part of a treatment for arthritis. If you are constipated, molasses acts as a mild natural laxative, stimulating better bowel function. This laxative effect is most useful in those with sluggish systems. It is not addictive, nor does your bowel become 'lazy' if you take molasses on a long-term daily basis.

Molasses has been shown in a scientific study to benefit the digestive system by encouraging the growth of healthy bacteria.[8] The study showed that molasses can be used effectively as a prebiotic because of the increase in healthy bacterial counts, which consequently inhibits the growth of pathogenic (disease-causing) bacteria. Molasses also normalizes the acidity level of the colon, therefore ensuring effective digestive function.

All the minerals and nutrients of unsulphured (organic) blackstrap molasses are in their natural, balanced form, creating a nutritional synergy that is difficult to find from supplements. These naturally abundant, nutrient-rich foods are worth their weight in gold for the health benefits they provide.

Directions

Molasses can be taken directly off the spoon at a maximum dose of 3 teaspoons daily. It can also be mixed into a little warm water and drunk immediately, or it can be used in cooking. Some people prefer to use molasses in their cider vinegar drinks (see earlier section on cider vinegar). Use 1 teaspoon in each glass.

• For an arthritis treatment programme, take 1 teaspoon three times daily.
• For a laxative effect, take 1–3 teaspoonfuls on an empty stomach.
• For anaemia, take 1 teaspoon three times daily, with or without food.
• For vegans and vegetarians wishing to maintain iron levels, take 2 teaspoons daily.
• To relieve daily fatigue and lack of concentration, take between 1 and 3 teaspoons daily, dependent on severity.

Green superfoods and alkaline minerals

We all know the age-old health philosophy, 'Eat your greens'. This may be an old-fashioned saying, but it still very much applies to modern health and we are finding out more and more about the reasons why green foods are so good for us.

Green foods and plants are particularly rich in a substance called chlorophyll. This substance is responsible for the green colour of plants. It is useful for health reasons due to its ability to oxygenate the body. Chlorophyll is quite remarkable in that its molecular structure is almost identical to our body's haemoglobin (found in red blood cells). The difference is that haemoglobin contains iron, whereas chlorophyll contains magnesium in its place. As we have seen, magnesium in itself is a beneficial alkaline mineral to people with arthritis but chlorophyll has other qualities aside from this. Chlorophyll is to plants what red blood cells are to us humans. Because of this similarity, chlorophyll can act in a similar way to haemoglobin in our bodies and help enrich our blood. Often associated with arthritis is anaemia, a deficiency of red blood cells. People with chronic inflammation in the body may take iron supplements for many years to no avail. However, chlorophyll may help in such cases to restore a healthier blood count.

The diverse benefits of chlorophyll

Chlorophyll is thought to have the ability to regenerate our health via cleansing, promoting detoxification, alkalizing, improving the quality of blood, and strengthening the immune system. Interestingly, there has been a great deal of research into its ability to prevent cancer and deal with the toxins within our system that may otherwise ultimately lead to cancer.

Dietary sources of chlorophyll

Green vegetables are the dietary source of chlorophyll. There is no absolute rule here as to which ones you use. It is however advantageous to vary the types you eat, bearing in mind the fact that the darker green varieties generally contain a higher proportion of chlorophyll.

Steaming vegetables for a short period of time is a better way to prepare them than boiling them in water and may even increase the amount of chlorophyll in a form that is readily taken into the body. Some, if not most, of the chlorophyll within the vegetables will be lost when boiling, especially for a long period of time. Eating a combination of raw green vegetables and lightly steamed variations should be the most reliable way to ensure the rich intake of chlorophyll.

Some examples to eat raw:

spinach
celery
lettuce
watercress
green peppers
green cabbage
olives
cucumber
herbs such as parsley, basil, fennel, mint and coriander.

And to steam:

broccoli
cabbage
kale
asparagus
Brussels sprouts
green beans
peas
chard
sea vegetables.

As well as chlorophyll, these foods all have the additional benefits of high vitamin and mineral content, alkaline properties, mild hormone-balancing activity, fibre content and antioxidant value. There are many reasons to eat a diet rich in green vegetables!

Easy greens . . . the supplements

Diet is one of the major ways to rebalance the acid/alkaline state of the body tissues. However, there are ways in which this process can be speeded up, by providing a concentrated amount of alkalizing minerals or substances on a daily basis in addition to following these dietary principles.

As little as a teaspoon of these powdered products can provide a huge amount of the nutrients found in greens, with all the nutrients and chlorophyll retained as far as is possible. It is effectively a cheat's way of obtaining nutrients, but when one has arthritis, it can be very difficult to buy, prepare and cook a variety of health-giving foods. If someone is eating a limited basic diet due to their state of health, then this type of product will be very useful as it will still provide the nutrients.

There are products available that provide these foods in their condensed form and retain powerful alkalizing properties. These can be added into the programme as a dietary supplement. Such products usually provide a good source of protein and calcium alongside the trace nutrients. Normally these are called 'Greens' and consist of a combination of one or more of the following alkaline superfoods:

alfalfa
nettle
aloe vera
spirulina
wheatgrass

barley grass
parsley
fennel
seaweed
algae
green tea leaves.

In addition to providing chlorophyll, the green superfoods also possess the following benefits:

- They increase energy levels.
- They cleanse and detoxify the body.
- They are a good source of protein, amino acids, enzymes, vitamins and minerals.
- They rebalance the acid/alkaline state of the body, thereby offering protection against cancer, arthritis, inflammatory disorders and many chronic diseases.
- They enhance nutrient intake, even for people who are debilitated and bed bound.

There are many variations on the super green products. Here's what to look for when buying:

- Search out fresh freeze-dried herbs, grasses, sea or freshwater greens. The process of fresh freeze-drying ensures that the maximum level of nutrients is preserved.
- Make sure green products are from an organic source to avoid contamination with pesticides, fertilizers and other frequently used toxic chemicals.
- Make sure they are free from additives, particularly those that try to conceal the taste, as this will diminish the quality of the product.
- A combination product rather than a single green product will provide more variation of nutrients and may produce better results.

Research was done to investigate the effect of diet on patients with rheumatoid arthritis.[9] Chlorophyll-rich juice was one of the two major components of the dietary changes made and the outcome was extremely positive. The diet not only decreased the symptoms of rheumatoid arthritis, but reduced the need for gold injections, methotrexate and steroids. The power of diet can be remarkable when you eat the right foods for your condition.

4

Category 2:
joint repair nutrients

The second category of supplements comprises the 'raw materials' for joint recovery. Without them, treating arthritis would be like trying to make a fabulous dinner without all the ingredients that the recipe requires. Specific nutrients can help repair damaged joints and the surrounding tissues. Without these, even if you are taking the supplements to relieve inflammation and pain, as well as alkalizing your body, it is unlikely that you will be able to achieve long-term benefit.

Now that we have considered steps to alkalizing the body, the next part of the programme is to supply nutrients that are capable of physically repairing joints. Addressing the acid/alkaline balance is of course crucial to success, but in the meantime there will be one or more damaged joints that need fast action to prevent further degeneration.

This is not easy to achieve – once a joint is in an arthritic state, its ability to repair itself is seriously impaired. The correct nutrients must be supplied via the diet and supplement products to restart and improve this crucial repair process.

The nutrients discussed in this chapter include broad spectrum multivitamins and minerals, protein supplements and popular products such as glucosamine and chondroitin.

Combination products: multivitamin and mineral formulas

The first step to ensuring an adequate nutrient supply to the affected joint, and to the body as a whole, is to correct any underlying dietary deficiencies. Of course, your diet itself should be as good as possible under the circumstances but a multinutrient formula may help to cover any possible 'gaps' in your nutritional intake. The intended use of such products is to be 'supplementary' to the diet rather than take the place of it. However, when people have poor mobility and are in varying degrees of pain, these ideals do not necessarily apply as the requirement for extra nutrients is simply too high.

Multivitamins are the products people tend to buy when they need something but they don't know what. They appear to cover all the bases and 'can't do any harm', so we tend to take them routinely. It is useful to have a product that covers all the potential underlying deficiencies that may have contributed to your condition. However, often such products contain small amounts of many nutrients rather than a sufficient dose of the ones you need and are therefore a waste of time and money. There are a few good combination formulas out there, though; the following information should help you to find them.

It is important to study the label to find out how much is provided of all of the active ingredients. This is the crucial aspect of choosing the right supplement. Ingredients are often listed as an amount in milligrams (mg) or micrograms (mcg or µg), followed by a % RDA value. The latter is very misleading as the RDA, the Recommended Daily Allowance, is not applicable to most situations. The RDA was developed during the Second World War as a means of setting the limits on the minimum intake requirements for essential nutrients to prevent a deficiency state. For example, such a deficiency state might have been scurvy, the disease associated with a vitamin C deficiency. Preventing such a deficiency is obviously important, but RDAs did not cover what was needed for optimum health and only accounted for healthy individuals – not those who might have a health problem. The RDA is often criticized within nutrition circles as being irrelevant and outdated.

If you have a disease of any sort, generally speaking, your nutrient requirements go up. Your body must work harder than a healthy body to achieve the same end result. Therefore if you were to consume only your RDA, then you would be unlikely to achieve success. You would need far more nutrients than the RDA accounts for.

On the label of a good-quality potent multivitamin supplement you may see % RDA values as high as 2,000–3,000 per cent. Do not let this alarm you, as this amount is what may be necessary to achieve good health. A good product will be well balanced, so when it provides high levels of one nutrient it will contain other nutrients to balance out the intake.

As a guide, a good basic formulation would include the nutrients listed in Table 1. I have given the various names under which you may find these listed on the label. Take particular note of the dose, as this is where the products can vary enormously.

Table 1: Recommended amounts of nutrients in a multivitamin supplement

Nutrient	Dose
B vitamin group:	
B1 (thiamine, thiamine HCL)	50 mg
B2 (riboflavin)	50 mg
B3 (niacin, niacinamide)	50–100 mg
B5 (pantothenic acid, calcium pantothenate)	50–500 mg
B6 (pyridoxine HCL)	50–100 mg
B9 folic acid (folate)	200–400 mg
B12 (cyanocobalamin)	25–400 µg
Vitamin C (ascorbic acid, calcium ascorbate)	200–500 mg
Selenium (selenomethionine)	50–200 µg
Vitamin A (retinyl palmitate, beta carotene)	1500 µg or 5000 iu
Vitamin D (cholecalciferol)	10–25 µg or 400–1000 iu
Vitamin E (natural rather than synthetic, α-tocopherol or mixed tocopherols)	200–800 iu

Unit measurements key: mg: milligram, µg: microgram, iu: international unit

There may be other ingredients such as kelp (to provide iodine and trace minerals), bioflavonoids, zinc, chromium, calcium, magnesium, Vitamin K, choline, inositol, manganese, iron, copper, etc. The table includes only the absolutely fundamental inclusions for a multinutrient formula.

Although they are basic nutritional components, the ability of vitamins and minerals to correct disease processes should never be underrated. Often in the health industry, a novel agent may be discovered that is surrounded by a great deal of hype. Because of these developments, people tend to forget about the basics and bypass the use of vitamins and minerals in favour of these new nutrients.

The first point of call should be to correct any potential deficiencies of the nutrients that naturally occur in the body and those that have a specific purpose. What follows is a summary of the main actions and facts about some of these important nutrients in relevance to arthritis and to general health.

Vitamin A

Vitamin A is crucial for eye health. It maintains the health of all the mucous membranes in the body, for example the lining of the digestive tract and lungs. The lining of the digestive tract is often adversely affected by medicines for arthritis. Many people with arthritis have anaemia, possibly due to the level of inflammation in the body; vitamin A helps to prevent anaemia, or corrects existing anaemia.

Vitamin A helps cells reproduce normally, preventing defects that may lead to illness. It supports strong immunity. Improper immune function can cause the onset of certain types of arthritis such as rheumatoid arthritis. It is required for normal development of the foetus and healthy reproduction, including the health of the placenta, sperm and ovaries. Fertility and pregnancy are often a concern in younger females with arthritis, as the medication used can seriously affect their ability to conceive and maintain a healthy pregnancy.

B vitamins

These are needed for DNA synthesis (which is the basis of all body cells). All cells contribute to the acid/alkaline balance of the body. Fatigue is a common issue among those with arthritis; B vitamins are crucial to a properly functioning metabolism, converting protein, fats and carbohydrates into energy.

B vitamins also support mental function and stress reduction. Coping with a normal daily routine can be very difficult for someone with arthritis, and those with arthritis often find their level of stress is increased due to frustration about their capabilities. Supporting the nervous system through such stress with B vitamins is very beneficial. They can have an antidepressant action, preventing an individual's physical condition from impacting on his or her mental health. They have anti-allergy potential. They also help in the formation of blood and prevent anaemia, often associated with arthritis.

B vitamins are often deficient among vegans and vegetarians. Taking them as a B complex rather than on their own enhances their action and maintains a good balance within the body.

Note that B vitamins are often depleted by medications. They are useful to take alongside medications and also afterwards once the drugs have been discontinued.

Vitamin C

An important antioxidant, Vitamin C is crucial when there is an increased level of inflammation in the body. It promotes the absorption of iron from food, preventing the occurrence of anaemia. It supports strong immune defences, keeping the immune system in balance to normalize autoimmune activity that leads to the forms of the condition seen in rheumatoid arthritis. It acts as a natural anti-histamine, relieving the strain on the immune system of those affected by seasonal or other allergies.

Vitamin C supports the health of the entire cardiovascular system. This is very important for those with rheumatoid arthritis as it tends to affect the entire body and the heart may be involved in complications of the disease. It may also help to reduce cholesterol. It supports adrenal function and therefore improves resistance to stress, a factor that can trigger or worsen arthritic symptoms and flare-ups.

Vitamin C requires bioflavonoids for its optimal functioning. These are usually derived from a citrus source and good vitamin C supplements often include such a source in their formulation.

Vitamin D

Vitamin D is very important for bone health and calcium metabolism; a report in 2010 stated that men with a deficiency of Vitamin D are twice as likely to have osteoarthritis of the hip.[1] Vitamin D is often deficient in the UK, especially northern areas where there is limited sunlight throughout the year as the vitamin is produced when the skin is exposed to natural sunlight. Your level of vitamin D can be tested by blood sample: 25-OHD or 25-hydroxyvitamin D. GPs can provide this service.

Sunscreens block the production of Vitamin D – the 'safe-sun' policy of use of sunscreens is thought to be partly responsible for the current widespread deficiency of vitamin D. Vitamin D is produced when skin is exposed to the sun for 20 to 30 minutes. Hence, it makes sense to allow this short period of sun exposure without sunscreen or too much covering up, while taking care not to redden or burn your skin.

Vitamin D supports immune function and may help resistance to influenza viruses. Keeping as well as possible through your arthritis treatment should be considered important to prevent setbacks caused by viral or bacterial infections. Evidence indicates a significant association of vitamin D deficiency with increased frequency of several auto-immune diseases (for example rheumatoid arthritis) and some cancers.[2]

Vitamin D may have antidepressant actions. It also plays a part in blood sugar control, useful for diabetes.

Vitamin E

An important antioxidant, Vitamin E is crucial for when inflammation is active or is increased in the body, and may protect joints from damage caused by inflammation as well as reducing pain.

It is an anti-blood clotting agent which may help to prevent thrombosis. The lack of mobility due to pain and stiffness may carry an increased risk of developing blood clots, caused by poor blood flow and consistency. Vitamin E dilates blood vessels and maintains the health of the arteries and veins, helping to prevent atherosclerosis (the furring up of arteries).

Vitamin E also supports the immune system and prevents premature ageing. It supports fertility and the health of the reproductive system, crucial for those with arthritis who are of childbearing age.

Selenium

The trace mineral selenium is crucial for thyroid function. An underactive thyroid can cause significant weight gain, tiredness, sluggishness and depression, all of which will impact on your arthritis. As an antioxidant, it works with Vitamin E and C. Selenium is especially likely to be deficient in cases of rheumatoid arthritis. Supplementation may help reduce pain and inflammation.

Calcium

Calcium is an abundant alkaline mineral that builds and maintains healthy bones and teeth. Osteoporosis is often considered a condition brought about by excess acid in the body, as alkaline minerals such as calcium are drawn out of the bone to neutralize the acid. Calcium may also be deficient in post-menopausal women, and medicines may deplete calcium levels.

Calcium requires a number of different nutrients – such as vitamin D, magnesium, vitamin K, boron and phosphorus – to be present alongside it if good bone health is to be achieved. Nutrients that operate together in this way are known as co-factors. Providing these minerals through the diet and supplements helps to protect the long-term health of the bone structure of the body.

Calcium is involved in muscle contraction, including the heart – the body's most important muscle. It also supports the normal functioning of the nervous system.

Hopefully what I have just said illustrates the importance of these basic nutrients. Each individual vitamin and mineral has far more functions in the body than those listed but further description would be too long for the purposes of this chapter.

If you have an inflammatory condition such as arthritis, you are also likely to be deficient in vitamins and minerals. The same applies if you are under stress, over-exercising, or have a poor or unvaried diet. Elderly people, pregnant women, anyone with chronic or acute illness, people with mobility restrictions and those who do not get outdoors enough are all at risk of nutrient deficiency. Unfortunately, due to today's eating habits and routines, most people of all ages could be described as nutrient depleted.

Protein foods

Protein is of fundamental importance in recovery from arthritis. It is often referred to as the 'elixir of life', and as its two main functions are growth and repair, you can see why. Arthritic joints are damaged or distressed joints, so they require a good deal of repair. Daily requirements for protein are much increased and a protein supplement is a suitable and convenient way to meet the body's increased demands.

A 2007 article published in a rheumatology journal stated that 'Progression of joint damage is likely to result primarily from an imbalance between cartilage degradation and repair.'[3] Such research indicates that if the body cannot repair the cartilage quickly enough then joint damage will worsen. As one of the two dominant functions of protein is to provide raw material for repairing the body, protein supplements are capable of slowing the progression of joint damage.

Amino acids are the building blocks of protein and each type of protein contains a different combination of amino acids, making it unique. Not all amino acids can be manufactured within the body and therefore they must be obtained through dietary means. If you don't eat the right foods, you may become deficient in protein. So, what foods provide good quality protein?

Protein is found in foods such as eggs, meat, poultry, fish, dairy products, legumes, nuts and seeds. An excess of protein from meat, however, can cause acid to build up in the body, so the key to supplying the right kind of protein to support your joints is to eat a balanced diet of the less acid-forming proteins. From this list, the most beneficial will be fish, eggs, chicken, and the vegetarian sources: legumes, seeds and nuts.

Protein supplements

Taking protein in supplement form will increase your daily intake in order to meet your higher requirements. As well as its benefits to the arthritic joints, protein is useful in maintaining a healthy weight, particularly if weight loss has occurred through the progression of arthritis – a situation often seen in people with rheumatoid arthritis. Most protein supplements are easy for the body to absorb and utilize; hence they give a distinct advantage in cases of poor digestion or malabsorption, which causes food nutrients to be wasted. Protein also helps to restore good energy levels as it plays a part in maintaining healthy blood sugar control.

There are many types of protein supplement to choose from. I recommend powders rather than protein-enriched bars and other products, as these tend to have unwanted additional ingredients. Powders can be sprinkled on to food or mixed into cold drinks such as apple juice, skimmed milk or a milk substitute such as almond milk, rice milk or soya milk. Protein powders can also be stirred into hot food, such as porridge, once cooked. If the powder itself is heated, however, it will be somewhat damaged.

An alternative to protein powder when going on holiday is amino acid tablets or capsules. These are easier to take while away from home but they deliver a much smaller amount of protein, so several capsules are needed to achieve the required intake.

Protein 'isolate' forms are more suitable for people with arthritis than 'concentrate' forms, which are more applicable in sports training. Isolates are more extensively purified forms of protein, whereas concentrates still contain some carbohydrate and fibre within their composition, which lowers the actual protein content per serving.

Protein supplements come from a variety of original sources. Soya, whey, pea and hemp all form the basis of available products; however, soya and whey versions have been more extensively studied for their health benefits.

Soya isolate has been identified as:

- a useful vegetarian and vegan source of protein;
- containing phytosterols and isoflavones, plant compounds useful for lowering cholesterol and reducing menopausal symptoms;
- 'A key factor in prevention and even treatment of rheumatoid arthritis'[4] due to its ability to decrease the severity of arthritis symptoms.

Whey isolate has been identified as:

- having an even higher absorbability than soya;
- possibly increasing antioxidant levels within the body – an additional benefit to help reduce inflammation.

Note however that whey isolate is not suitable for vegetarians or vegans as it is a dairy product.

Dose

This will vary dependent on body weight and dietary protein intake, but a typically good product should provide between 8 and 16 grams of protein per daily serving.

Cautions

Anyone diagnosed with liver or kidney dysfunction should seek professional advice before taking protein or amino acid supplements. Protein supplements may interact with some medications, particularly those for Parkinson's disease.

Avoid supplements with artificial sweeteners or flavourings.

Nutritional supplements for joint repair

Nutritional supplements that directly provide substances found naturally within joints help to repair the joint and prevent further damage caused by arthritis. This is a crucial part of the recovery process. While it takes time for the symptoms of arthritis to diminish, in the meantime focus must be put on preserving the affected joints.

First, we will take a look at the inner workings of the joint. Understanding the function of the different components helps us to see why these supplements may help in symptom reduction:

Glossary of joint terms

Synovial fluid   A yolk-like fluid found in joint cavities. Its main functions are to reduce friction between the bones of the joint; supply nutrients and remove metabolic waste products from the joint; and act as a shock absorber – the fluid can change its thickness depending on the strain put on the joint. 'Synovitis' is the term used to describe when the fluid builds up within the joint and the surrounding membrane casing becomes inflamed. This is common in rheumatoid arthritis.

Cartilage   A type of connective tissue that serves as a cushion between the bones of the joints. It is made up of water and substances called proteoglycans and collagen.

Collagen   A mesh of protein fibres found in connective tissue of joints/ cartilage. Arthritis is characterized by degradation of cartilage in the joints, causing pain and limited movement.

Proteoglycans   Protein structures found within cartilage. Proteoglycans interact with collagen to maintain the health of the cartilage.

Glycosaminoglycans   These are used to make proteoglycans, a major component of joint cartilage. Examples of glycosaminoglycans are glucosamine and chondroitin (see below).

Cartilage plays a crucial part in the progression of arthritis. In osteoarthritis, the cartilage wears away and becomes quite ragged and brittle. Bone beneath the cartilage responds by thickening slightly and producing an uneven roughened surface, which then makes the internal space between the two ends of the joint narrower. The bones eventually begin to rub against each other, producing pain and inflammation. Pieces of the degrading cartilage can break off and float around in the synovial fluid, causing more inflammation. Often small pieces of bone may also break away into the fluid space and cause the 'locking' of the joint that many people with arthritis will have experienced.

There are a number of reasons why degradation of the cartilage occurs, but most often it is nutrient deficiency or mechanical stress on the joint – from either being overweight or exercising improperly – that is the cause. Once the process starts, the joint subsequently suffers from the action of inflammatory substances and those which degrade the joint structures further.

Age is a factor in the development of joint problems. As we get older, the amount of proteoglycans in the cartilage decreases. As fewer and fewer proteoglycans are available, cartilage will start to degrade over time in the natural course of ageing. This is what we mean when we refer to arthritis as a condition of ageing or 'simply getting old'. Older people with arthritis may still be helped by the replenishment of all the raw materials that maintain the proteoglycans, the collagen and subsequently the cushioning cartilage itself.

The use of supplements based on supporting the cartilage and surrounding joint components not only helps reduce pain in some people but also seems to slow the degeneration of the arthritic joint. The following are the most widely used supplements:

Glucosamine A dietary supplement made up of basic sugars (glucose) and amino acids. It can preserve and regenerate cartilage, and support the structure and function of joints.

Chondroitin A dietary supplement. An important structural component of cartilage, it contributes to joint cushioning.

Hyaluronic acid Provides the lubrication of the joint and improves the viscosity of synovial fluid. It also helps assist the uptake of nutrients and water into the cartilage. It improves mobility and flexibility of the joint. It may also help dry, wrinkled skin. Until recently hyaluronic acid could only be obtained via injections administered at hospital, but it is now available as a dietary supplement.

If you use the nutrients mentioned above, it may commonly be several weeks before improvements are noticeable. As they are all based on altering the quality of the joint structures and fluid, this process is not going to be fast; a long-term course of therapy will be needed. But the effects of such joint nutrients seem to be long lasting, continuing well after the treatment has been discontinued. This makes it seem likely that these supplements are effective in permanently rebuilding and supporting the joint structures.

Some of the research relating to substances that affect the structural components of the joint is quite promising. In 2004, a *Current Drug Targets* study stated that chondroitin sulphate was capable of producing a 'slow but gradual decrease of the clinical symptoms of osteoarthritis and these benefits last for a long period after the end of treatment'.[5] This suggests that chondroitin sulphate not only works on reducing symptoms but that, in doing so, it is permanently altering the health of the knee structures, hence the lasting effect. The same study discussed the possibility that chondroitin sulphate could have anti-inflammatory effects and a chondroprotective (joint protecting) action.

The journal *Osteoarthritis Cartilage*, in 2008, stated that they 'definitely have enough clinical data available supporting the view that oral chondroitin sulphate is a valuable and safe symptomatic treatment for osteoarthritis disease'.[6] Safety is a primary concern, considering that many people with arthritis are being prescribed medications whose safety is questionable.

A 2009 study examined the effects of a combined product of glucosamine, chondroitin and quercetin and found it to be very beneficial for osteoarthritis, although not for rheumatoid arthritis.[7] After three months of treatment there was a significant improvement in pain symptoms and the ease with which daily activities (such as walking up and down stairs) could be performed. The researchers investigated the joints themselves and found beneficial effects on the synovial fluid.

A life sciences publication in 2009 made the following statement about chondroitin sulphate: 'Its effects include benefits that are not achieved by current medicines and include chondroprotection and the prevention of joint space narrowing. Such positive effects of chondroitin sulphate represent a breakthrough in the treatment of hip and knee OA.'[8]

A comparative study looked at glucosamine sulphate as an alternative to ibuprofen, a non-steroidal anti-inflammatory drug commonly prescribed for arthritic pain.[9] Over 170 patients were involved and the outcome was in favour of glucosamine, as it achieved reduction of symptoms as effectively as ibuprofen but without the side effects. The dose used within the study was 1,500 mg daily of glucosamine compared to 1,200 mg daily of ibuprofen. It was concluded that glucosamine is a good alternative therapy for osteoarthritis.

Studies in 2005 found hyaluronic acid injections to be effective for mild to severe cases of osteoarthritis, with the effects lasting up to 19 weeks after the injection was given.[10] Hyaluronic acid was most successful at decreasing disability level and permitting improved walking speed.

Additional considerations

Vitamin C is particularly important in the rebuilding of healthy collagen. Collagen will degrade if there is an insufficient supply of vitamin C to the joint, despite the availability of other nutrients. Always consider the use of a multinutrient formulation before trying the joint nutrient supplements mentioned here, as many of the vitamins and minerals are needed to facilitate these repair processes.

Cartilage has a limited ability to repair itself fully, but normally the health of the joint can be improved to some extent and the degradation halted by providing the correct nutrients and allowing adequate rest. The other joints in the body must be considered when one has arthritis in, for example, a knee. The knee may be beyond repair; however, the same process that caused the knee to degenerate may well be affecting other joints in the body, so no efforts to restore overall joint health would be wasted.

Food sources of glycosaminoglycans

Stock made from good quality chicken bones provides a rich source of these joint nutrients. It is now considered old-fashioned to make your own stock – most people use stock cubes. However, using stock you have made yourself can provide many benefits to your joints.

To the leftover carcass of a cooked chicken, add a stick of celery, a chopped onion, a chopped carrot, fresh or dried parsley, a bay leaf, a few peppercorns, and ½ tsp sea salt. Cover with water and bring to the boil. Reduce heat to a simmer and cook for about four hours, occasionally skimming off any foam that comes to the surface. Remove the bones and strain the stock. When cooled, pour the stock into ice cube trays or ice cube bags for freezing. To use the stock, use one to two cubes instead of a stock cube.

Use each time you make soup or cook rice, whenever you need stock. It makes a very tasty base for risottos, soups and sauces while helping your joints.

Recommended dose of supplements

• Glucosamine 1,500 mg daily, ideally in divided doses (i.e. throughout the day).

- Chondroitin 1,200 mg daily, again in divided doses.

Combination products are available which may have more potent effects than taking a singular supplement.

Cautions

Glucosamine

Glucosamine is sourced from shellfish; do not take it if you are allergic to shellfish. There is another source available known as vegetarian glucosamine (normally made from corn); however, this is not the type tested in most of the studies available.

Monitor your blood glucose levels frequently, as there is a theoretical link that supplementation may affect those with diabetes.

Glucosamine may cause gastrointestinal upset in sensitive individuals.

Chondroitin

Chondroitin is sourced from cow, pig or shark, and is therefore unsuitable for vegetarians or vegans. If you have a prostate disorder, you should seek professional advice before taking chondroitin. It may also have anti-blood clotting effects – consult your doctor if you are taking warfarin. And it may cause gastrointestinal upset in sensitive individuals.

Hyaluronic acid

Although this is now available in oral supplement form from health food stores, please note that the research mainly refers to injections of hyaluronic acid, rather than the tablet version.[11]

5

Category 3: supplements to relieve inflammation and pain

Although it is vital in the longer term to repair the damage caused by arthritis, the day-to-day symptoms, such as pain, stiffness, swelling and hot joints, and their associated restrictions on mobility, require action now, today. When you are suffering you need help immediately.

Inflammation can be dangerous, as well as being extremely uncomfortable and debilitating to live with. Supplements from Category 3 will make the journey to recovery much easier and even possibly quicker.

Natural solutions include nutritional supplements such as enzymes, antioxidants and herbal products to relieve the pain and inflammation of arthritis. Most can normally be used in conjunction with prescribed painkillers and anti-inflammatories. They generally take some time to become effective. By taking these natural products alongside your prescribed medications to begin with, you give yourself the best of both worlds as regards pain relief. It may be your intention to gradually withdraw from prescribed pain medications and this will be easier to cope with once such nutritional supplements begin to take effect.

Natural solutions for pain relief and reducing inflammation

The most inhibiting aspect of having arthritis is the pain and subsequent immobility it causes. If there is a way to somehow get this daily pain under more control, then transition to recovery will be much smoother and more easily accomplished.

Steroid injections, anti-inflammatories and other types of drugs can often have a strong effect on pain. But they have serious disadvantages, including both the long-term side effects of taking such medicines and the day-to-day side effects which can, for some people, be difficult to cope with. Not only is exploring natural options for control of pain much safer for the body, but the outcome can improve the underlying condition and enable recovery.

Most people who turn to natural methods of pain control do so because they find themselves in one of the following situations:

- They cannot tolerate any of the pharmaceutical medications, and so are unable to take a regular course of treatment.
- Their prescribed medication is ineffective at controlling their symptoms.
- They are currently getting on well with their medication but are worried about the long-term effects.
- They are simply inclined to find a way of supporting and improving their body's own pain relief systems.

I have yet to see anyone who is content to remain on strong medication indefinitely. Most people aspire to reduce or discontinue their medications and do not want to be on them 'for life'.

Generally speaking it is not wise to discontinue a drug suddenly; arthritis drugs are very potent and strong acting so to stop taking them altogether would likely cause a massive flare-up of your condition. If it is your intention to eventually stop taking prescription drugs, it is important to do so by gradually reducing the dose, ideally under the supervision of a consultant who can monitor your progress and perform various tests to ensure a safe, smooth transition.

Consultants may support your decision to discontinue arthritis medicines, or they may not. Practitioners within their field do not always know or believe that there are alternative ways of dealing with arthritis, or that in fact it is possible to recover completely in some cases. They are understandably reluctant to reduce medication as they are not confident that their patient will improve without the drugs. However, more often than not, once the drugs are out of a person's system, the results from a natural treatment programme become far more marked. Some people experience dramatic improvements in their health after discontinuing their medicines. It must be done responsibly though – slowly, little by little.

I would suggest that you spend at least a month or two on a natural treatment programme before considering any changes at all to your medication. Your body needs to stabilize with each change you make and supplements usually help to achieve this more effectively. Without taking supplements and making necessary dietary changes, it can be too difficult or even perhaps detrimental to stop taking prescribed medicines.

Nutrition can be powerful for relieving pain and calming inflammation. As different substances affect pain and inflammation in different ways, they can be divided into five groups each offering a different treatment option – all are invaluable.

1 *Endorphins*, the body's own pain-reducing chemicals. Amino acids, such as DLPA (see p. 56), enable these chemicals to work to the best of their ability. DLPA increases the body's production of endorphins which act to reduce pain.
2 *Antioxidants*, such as Vitamin E, soak up excessive amounts of dangerous free radicals: harmful molecular substances that are produced when the body is in a state of inflammation.
3 *Enzymes*, when taken on an empty stomach, have an anti-inflammatory action and other effects such as improving the circulation. This helps the transport of nutrients and clearance of toxins or waste matter.
4 *Fats* within the body can be out of balance and wreak havoc. The right fats, or fatty acids, are beneficial and have an anti-inflammatory action; the wrong fats cause inflammation.
5 *Herbal compounds* such as ginger can be used in either a dietary or supplement form. Herbs can be broad acting – they have more than one effect on pain, inflammation and joint health in general.

Options 2 and 3 are particularly useful to limit the amount of damage caused by arthritis, whereas options 1 and 5 may be exceptionally useful for controlling the day-to-day pain you experience. Option 4 is an essential part of the full recovery process, as it corrects one of the possible contributors to chronic inflammation.

Please note that the options described are generally (but not always) slower acting than conventional, prescribed medications; however, they tend to have a much longer lasting effect as they are correcting body imbalances along the way. We will now take an in-depth look at these five options.

Endorphins – the body's internal pain relief system

Endorphins are the body's natural painkillers. They are a group of naturally occurring compounds that can have a powerful pain-reducing effect. Produced within all of our bodies, these natural painkillers are dependent on the good functioning of our nervous system. Endorphins work in a similar way to morphine, a strong pain-relieving medication. They are thought to block pain receptors in the brain and spinal cord;

therefore, when pain is present somewhere in your body they ensure that your conscious awareness of this pain is very much reduced. Any way of increasing the activity of these substances should be beneficial to those with chronic pain.

One factor that hugely impacts on the body's natural production of pain chemicals is stress. At different times in our lives we are subjected to stress of various types: unrelenting physical work, family or relationship worries, mental efforts such as exams, emotional stress such as anxiety. Most people with arthritis notice that when a stressful event or situation occurs in their lives, the pain of their arthritis usually flares up, or their recovery is very much impaired. Under normal circumstances, the brain releases endorphins as part of the normal physiological response to stress. But, like every system in the body, if it is overworked it eventually tires and its ability to carry out this function slows down. So, when stress is constant and unrelenting, inadequate endorphins are produced as the supply simply runs out. The person then becomes much less tolerant of pain – her pain threshold is lowered. Chronic pain is a huge stress in itself and impairs the body in the way that I have just described. When pain relief is needed most, the body cannot stand up to its demands and the condition worsens. This happens commonly in arthritis.

Option 1: Restoring endorphin levels for natural pain relief

The body's natural endorphins are thought to be fifty or so times more effective than morphine in terms of pain relief. We often take painkillers such as morphine, codeine, dihydrocodeine and tramadol when we are in severe pain. However, when taken repeatedly they may cause dependence and unpleasant side effects. If we can find a safe but reliable way to improve the body's ability to produce and utilize its natural painkillers, it should be extremely beneficial to those struggling to cope with the debilitating chronic pain from arthritis. So let us now consider what nutrients are needed to support this process and help it work efficiently so that pain is markedly reduced.

Adequate dietary protein Endorphins are made up of many amino acids, the constituents of protein, which need to be present in sufficient quantities in the body. When you are in extreme chronic pain on a daily basis, your diet may be insufficient in protein among other nutrients – it is simply too much effort to prepare food or even eat at all. A good diet must be encouraged. However, you can and should use a protein supplement to further improve your intake (see section on protein supplements in Chapter 4).

Extra nutrients   These are needed to support the body when under the stress of chronic pain; without them endorphins will become depleted. Such nutrients include vitamin B complex, zinc, magnesium, vitamin C and DLPA.

Most of these nutrients are discussed in other sections of the book. However, DLPA is a very different type of nutrient and I will explain its remarkable effects here.

  DLPA, otherwise known as DL-phenylalanine, is a nutrient that helps to restore the levels of endorphins, the body's natural painkillers. It is an amino acid that has a direct effect on the physiology of the brain's receptors for pain. It prevents a particular enzyme from destroying endorphins, the morphine-like substances that naturally occur in our nervous systems to provide our bodies with an internal source of pain relief. By blocking this enzyme, DLPA actually increases the amount of endorphins. These active, circulating, naturally occurring chemicals then become more abundant and produce a pain-relieving effect for longer.

  Leon Chaitow, in his book *Amino Acids in Therapy*, states that DLPA does not act as an analgesic (painkilling) tablet, but rather allows the body's own internal pain control mechanism to act in a more advantageous manner.[1] Chaitow discusses research that indicates the achievement of rapid and lasting pain relief from both rheumatoid and osteoarthritis.

  It can take a while to feel the benefits of using DLPA. Often people report that it has taken several weeks to produce a good level of pain relief but that it does work, given the opportunity. If DLPA is used in conjunction with nutrients that support the nervous system, there is a far better chance of an overall reduction in pain.

- DLPA is thought to produce pain relief that lasts for up to five days, very long lasting compared to most pain relief medicines.
- DLPA has anti-inflammatory as well as pain-relieving properties. Endorphins block the activity of prostaglandins – other natural chemicals that produce inflammation.
- Its effects tend to be stronger over time, i.e. the longer it is taken, the better the pain relief obtained.

- DLPA is thought to have antidepressant qualities due to its beneficial effects on brain chemicals.
- Unlike morphine and other drugs that modulate the endorphins in the brain, DLPA is *not* addictive even when taken long term. There is a natural system in the brain that prevents it becoming addicted to its own internal endorphins and natural manipulation of this system by DLPA will not produce an addiction.[2]

Cautions and contraindications

DLPA is not suitable for those with the genetic condition PKU (phenyl-ketonuria), as such people cannot metabolize phenylalanine correctly. It may not be suitable for those with hypertension (high blood pressure), although it should not interfere if taken after food.

Option 2: Antioxidants

Antioxidants are often mentioned in health circles, and in newspapers and magazines, and many products claim to contain high levels of these nutrients. However, it is not widely understood why antioxidants are so good for us and what they actually do in the body.

Considering this subject in the context of inflammatory diseases, we find that inflammation within the body goes hand in hand with a process called oxidation.[3] This is when free molecules of oxygen react with other free molecules; in combination, these newly formed molecular substances are extremely damaging to the cells and tissues of the body. This process is thought to be associated with many conditions including premature ageing, Alzheimer's disease, diabetes, liver and kidney disease and arthritis.

An example of the everyday occurrence of the oxidation process is the browning of an apple once its flesh is exposed to air. This is essentially the same process that occurs biologically within our bodies. If lemon juice is added to the flesh of the apple, it will prevent it from browning. This is due to the content of vitamin C (ascorbic acid) within the lemon, which acts as an antioxidant. If there is no vitamin C present then the apple will brown quickly. Use this to visualize what is happening within the body of a person with arthritis: a lot of oxidation is taking place, more so than in a healthy person, and each reaction drains the body's supply of anti-oxidants. Antioxidant supplies gradually drain away, and if they are not replenished, further damage and degeneration of the joints occurs.

There are ways to prevent this type of damage. One is to increase the intake of dietary antioxidants found in the foods we consume. Fresh, seasonal food will be rich in antioxidants. However, in processed food, the amounts present may be extremely low or even non-existent. Current issues such as high food miles, the methods we use to preserve food and the unavailability of foods in season can all also degrade the quality of the food we are eating. The outcome is that many people succumb to dietary deficiencies.

Antioxidants are present in varying amounts in many fruits and vegetables, in herbs, spices and nuts, and in many other foods. Coloured fruits and vegetables are especially high in antioxidants and the best advice is to include within your alkaline diet foods of as many different colours as possible, as this will provide you with a wide variety of different types of antioxidants that may all have slightly differing benefits. Foods that can be incorporated to benefit your arthritis include:

broccoli
Brussels sprouts
cauliflower
apples
pears
peaches
apricots
pumpkin
squash
red, green and yellow peppers
sweet potato
beetroot
kale
spinach
onions
dark green vegetables
nuts
nut butters
avocados
sunflower and pumpkin seeds
oatmeal
legumes (beans, lentils, peas)
wholegrains

herbs such as turmeric, cloves, cinnamon and ginger
green tea.

Antioxidants and our internal defence mechanism

Major antioxidant enzymes built into our bodies protect us from damage. One example is called superoxide dismutase (SOD). Researchers found that the cartilage in the joints of those with osteoarthritis was significantly deficient in superoxide dismutase, the major antioxidant enzyme.[4] This enzyme relies on adequate amounts of zinc and copper for its functioning and without these present in sufficient quantity it cannot perform its antioxidant duties. Therefore zinc and copper are two very important nutrients to support the body's own antioxidant defence system. Other antioxidant nutrients include the following:

vitamin C
vitamin E
selenium
beta carotene
astaxanthin
pycnogenol
coQ10
resveratrol
bioflavonoids
zinc
copper
amino acids, especially cysteine, glutamine and taurine
manganese
magnesium.

Antioxidant nutrients tend to work better when they are taken in combination rather than in isolation. A mixed antioxidant product containing several of the above nutrients should be more effective than taking, for example, vitamin C on its own. To illustrate the way in which these substances interact with each other, vitamin E actually recycles vitamin C so that it can be used again and again as an antioxidant. So you will gain more benefit from vitamin C if it is combined with vitamin E.

Combined supplements are available in health food shops; they may be needed in addition to a balanced diet to reliably obtain a broad spectrum of antioxidant nutrients. Remember to start with a varied diet – do not be tempted to neglect this in favour of supplements. Use these in addition to the diet rather than as substitutes for healthy eating.

A look at some of the research shows well-documented effects of several types of antioxidants on the prevention, treatment and progression of arthritis. In particular, there is strong focus on rheumatoid arthritis. Antioxidants seem to be more advantageous here than in osteoarthritis, the degenerative type of arthritis, although they may still help to some extent.

- The *Journal of Medicinal Food* observed the effects of vitamin E and quercetin on the level of inflammation and found a positive outcome.[5] It concluded that a dietary deficiency of vitamin E increased the inflammatory response and that using antioxidants to treat inflammation was successful.
- Collagen is crucial to the development and maintenance of muscle, cartilage, tendon, and bone structure. Arthritis patients who had high vitamin C intakes decreased their risk of disease progression by 300 per cent.[6]
- Vitamin E can reduce osteoarthritis-induced pain, and also helps to build cartilage.[7]
- A different study in *Annals of the Rheumatic Diseases* found that a low antioxidant level is a risk factor for developing rheumatoid arthritis. The antioxidants measured in this case were vitamin E, beta-carotene and selenium.[8]
- A 2009 study found grapeseed extract to be potentially very useful in the treatment of rheumatoid arthritis via its actions as an antioxidant.[9]
- An interesting piece of research was done on patients who were taking the drug methotrexate and added to their therapy the antioxidant coQ10. They found that the coQ10 potentiated the effect of methotrexate, i.e. helped it work better, and that it had anti-arthritic action as well as its known properties as an antioxidant.[10]
- Research suggests that bioflavonoids reduce pain and inflammation.[11]

Option 3: Enzymes

Enzymes are miracle workers in the body with many varying functions. These complex protein molecules reduce inflammation, reduce pain and improve circulation. They break down food and help its conversion into energy, support immune function and help the liver detoxify. Their specific action depends on timing, i.e. when they are taken. When taken on an empty stomach they alleviate the pain and inflammation of arthritis. When taken with food, they work on improving digestion.

If taken on an empty stomach, when there is no food to digest, enzymes become absorbed into the systemic circulation of the body where they work on inflammation. If taken with food, enzymes assist the breakdown of that food. Although the latter may be useful for some, this will not help with the relief of pain and inflammation.

There are many different enzymes; some are single enzymes and some are combinations of four or five different enzymes, each with a slightly different function. Fresh fruit and vegetables, of course, contain their own enzymes that aid digestion of that food. Enzymes are also present in seeds, nuts and sprouted grains. They are mostly destroyed by cooking or heating.

Deficiencies in enzymes are common, largely due to our diet but also due to the lack of essential vitamins and minerals that are needed to activate the enzymes and make them work correctly. Many different enzymes in the body rely on a supply of zinc. A mild to moderate deficiency of zinc is common in contemporary society, due in part to our intensive farming methods and food processing industry. Zinc deficiency also seems to be extremely common in those with arthritis of any type, illustrating the need to correct such deficiencies to enable our own enzymes to work effectively again.

People who are deficient in, for example, digestive enzymes will experience gastrointestinal disease. They may experience symptoms such as bloating, gas, abdominal pains and low energy levels.

Restoring good enzyme function throughout the entire body will improve the health of an individual on countless levels as enzymes have so many diverse uses. All of the body's systems and processes rely on the good functioning of enzymes.

How do enzymes work to alleviate arthritis?

As you can see, enzymes have many functions within the body. But how do they relieve the pain and inflammation of arthritis? They are thought to act in various ways to do this:

- by inhibiting the production of pain chemicals in the body;
- by digesting and breaking down damaged tissue while sparing healthy tissue, thereby helping to clear debris from within the joint;
- by speeding up the repair of damaged areas and also helping to clear excess fluids, i.e. swelling, from the joint.

These actions can all be achieved by using enzyme supplements. They can be either from a plant or animal source. Animal sources generally provide three different types of enzymes that digest protein, starch and fat; however, plant sources provide an even wider range of enzymes, which maximizes their chance of being effective. Whether you are using plant- or animal-based enzymes, you should always take them between meals to allow them to achieve their anti-inflammatory effect.

A research study was performed on enzyme supplements, comparing their effects to diclofenac, a prescribed anti-inflammatory drug commonly given for pain relief for arthritis.[12] It found that the enzyme formula was a safe and effective alternative to diclofenac when treating osteoarthritis of the knee.

All enzymes should benefit your arthritis. The following are types that have been more widely tested for their pain-relieving and anti-inflammatory effects:

Bromelain   Found in pineapples. (Although the fruit itself is not recommended as part of the diet for arthritis, the enzyme within it is very useful to use in a supplement.)

Papain   Found in papaya fruit.

Protease   An enzyme that digests proteins in the body.

Serrapeptase   A specific type of protease.

When looking for a product, see if it contains one or more of these enzymes. Otherwise choose a broad-spectrum digestive enzyme formula.

Reading the labels, you will see that the quantity of each enzyme is expressed both in milligrams (mg) and also as a unit value. For example, the label of a fat-digesting enzyme may read: 'Lipase 10mg/500 lipase units' (LUs). As the unit value and milligrams vary depending on the type of enzyme, it is not possible to advise you how many units to look for in a specific product. Do, however, use the guidelines given in the example below for how to take the product and start with a low dose, only increasing it if you need more relief of your symptoms.

Serrapeptase

Here is an example of a unique type of enzyme called serrapeptase, which I have seen achieve good results among people with pain from arthritis. Serrapeptase is an enzyme derived from the silkworm. It is produced by the silkworm in order to digest its cocoon due to its ability to break down proteins. Serrapeptase, as a supplement, is thought to have many unique effects, mainly in dealing with inflammation in the body. It is, therefore, appropriate to use for many conditions and to my knowledge, it has no reported side effects whatsoever. It is considered an entirely safe supplement.

These effects have not been widely researched. However, in my experience it has proven successful in many different cases of arthritis. Osteoarthritic pain tends to respond faster to this enzyme therapy than rheumatoid arthritis, which, although still achieving considerable benefit, appears to require more intensive treatment.

Dose

Although this is a guide to dosage of serrapeptase, you can use it as a guide for other enzyme supplements.

- For osteoarthritis – to reduce pain and inflammation take 1 capsule three times daily, between meals (i.e. it must be taken on an empty stomach). This dose can be increased if necessary.
- For rheumatoid arthritis – to reduce pain and inflammation, take up to 3 capsules at a time, three times daily between meals. In some cases, it may be appropriate to go to an even higher dose than this; however, the financial cost may prevent you from doing so.

Option 4: Essential fats – achieving the optimal balance

In the body there are many different types of fats, some good, some bad. All of these contribute to the level of inflammation in the body, whether by reducing it or promoting it. The fats that are considered bad – saturated and trans fats (see glossary on p. 70) for example – generally cause inflammation in the body if there is too much of them. The good fats, those rich in omega 3 for example, can counteract inflammation in the body. Increasing your intake of these beneficial fats can help to relieve your pain.

Why are the fats within our bodies so out of balance?

There is probably more discussion of fats than any other food group and many controversial statements are made about fats within the media, among weight loss groups and within medicine. Fats are reputed to be both pro-inflammatory and anti-inflammatory, to be involved in both weight gain and weight reduction; they are the subject of a myriad of confusing claims. In this section I will try to dispel some of the myths and help provide more understanding of how to use fats to benefit your arthritis.

Our food culture has changed very much over the last twenty years. We could now be described as a fat-phobic nation, with the typical Western diet providing a completely unbalanced supply of fats; less of the right type and more of the harmful. Many people are actively worsening the situation without realizing it as they eliminate beneficial fats from their diet, perhaps because they are trying to lose weight. Little do they know that they are upsetting the balance and leaving themselves more susceptible to inflammatory diseases by doing so.

This fat phobia is often encouraged by the many weight loss, fat-reducing diet plans available. Hundreds of fat-free and low-fat products, containing alternatives to fat, occupy space on supermarket shelves; foods that have been doctored to accommodate the huge market of people who believe fat makes you gain weight. The problem with the many diet schemes around is that they are very much open to interpretation or, perhaps too frequently, misinterpretation. It is true that some types of fat will cause weight gain. Some fats, however, actually help you to lose weight and correct your metabolism and bodily functions, thereby making you much healthier. These useful fats are known as the essential fatty acids. Essential simply means that these fats are not produced in sufficient quantities within the body, and so must be obtained from the diet.

Weight is often an issue among people with arthritis. Osteoarthritis, in particular, is thought to be aggravated when too much strain is placed on the joints through excess weight or obesity. Weight reduction is often part of programmes to treat arthritis – simply taking the physical pressure off the joints can help reduce symptoms of arthritis. Therefore, it is clear that the issue of fats can be a double-edged sword to those with arthritis. They need the fats more than ever to help their body normalize the level of inflammation; however, they may well be trying to lose weight by cutting out the very fats their body requires.

Many people take diets to the extreme, cutting out every type of fat even so far as to eliminate nuts, seeds, avocados and other beneficial fats and oils. To rely on a diet that includes no fats is unlikely to produce sustainable weight loss, although in some the calorie reduction and reduced portion size can cause a dramatic loss of weight. But it leaves the body in a much unhealthier state. This method of weight loss is usually followed by rebound weight gain shortly afterwards. The goal is never reached and this yo-yo pattern can continue for a great many years.

Of course, it must be said that an excess of saturated fats, particularly those from animal sources, and trans fats, such as those in margarines and many processed foods, is extremely detrimental. These fats should be removed from your diet whether you wish to lose weight or relieve your arthritis, or both. Your intake of 'good' fats, however, should be increased and, no matter what your starting weight is, should form a part of a healthy diet. Foods such as oily fish, nuts, seeds, avocados, some eggs and oils of walnut, flaxseed and hemp should frequently be present within daily meals. All of these foods contain some level of omega 3, one of the natural providers of essential fatty acids. This is the most anti-inflammatory of all the types of fats and ironically tends to be the type in which most of us are deficient if eating a typical Western diet.

Heating fats can become an issue. This is relevant mainly to the oils used in cooking but also refers to fats within foods that may reach a certain temperature when cooked. At high temperatures, many fats begin to lose their structure and can turn into what is known as a trans fat. These trans fats are the most detrimental to health as they are unnatural and can leave the body prone to inflammation. For cooking I would recommend using coconut oil, as this remains stable even when heated at very high temperatures. Coconut oil is quite high in saturated fat; however, it has many benefits to the body and therefore is thought to be a healthy fat. Coconut oil is rich in a substance called caprylic acid, a very effective anti-fungal. When taken regularly, it can benefit the balance of gut bacteria, helping to rid the body of harmful levels of yeasts and bacteria. For example, the condition candida albicans is an overgrowth of a type of yeast and is often present in people with arthritis; it is particularly prevalent among those with autoimmune types such as rheumatoid arthritis. You may also use olive oil for stir frying. It is best to avoid low-calorie spray alternatives to cooking oils, as these are highly processed; instead use sparing amounts of coconut or olive oil.

The balance of fats among people with arthritis is very commonly affected. Such an imbalance can promote inflammation in the body, whereas correction can have a potent anti-inflammatory effect, thereby relieving many of the symptoms of the arthritis. Getting this balance just right is crucial in enabling a person to recover well from arthritis.

In the context of diet and supplements, the main area we will focus on here is the beneficial essential fats, also known as essential fatty acids.

Dietary changes

Try to avoid the following fats:

- animal fats (in excess)
- trans fats (margarine, processed foods)
- low-fat substitutes
- saturated fats in excess (e.g. cream, butter).

Make sure you eat more of the polyunsaturated and monounsaturated fats found in oily fish (mackerel, wild salmon, sardines), nuts, seeds, avocados, flaxseed oil, walnut oil, hemp seeds and oil (see glossary on p. 70). Cook with coconut oil or olive oil.

Read the label

As you now know that not all fats are bad and some are very beneficial, it will be useful to familiarize yourself with the names of the types of fat as they are listed on the labels of food products. If a food is high in saturated fat, it should be avoided; on the other hand, a food high in polyunsaturated fat will be beneficial to you, at least from the point of view of its fat content. Monounsaturated fats, such as those found within olive oil and avocados, can also benefit you. See glossary at the end of this section for details of the types of fats.

Essential fatty acid supplements

The dietary advice given here will help you to some extent to correct the balance of fats in your system. However, when you have an inflammatory condition such as arthritis, you will gain a much more powerful benefit from taking fats in supplement form in addition to your diet.

For anti-inflammatory effects, a fish body oil is ideal. Its useful ingredients are EPA and DHA (see glossary on pp. 69–70). These are naturally occurring compounds that have been shown in several scientific studies to reduce inflammation in the body.

In terms of beneficial levels of these substances, a product containing about 750 mg of EPA and 500 mg of DHA should be sufficient to provide an anti-inflammatory effect, although you may find you need a little more than this. A high potency product may contain as much as 2,000 mg of EPA and 1,500 mg of DHA per daily intake.

Flaxseed oil is a vegan source of omega 3 fats. However, as it is sourced from a plant, it is much more difficult for your body to obtain the required dose to enable an anti-inflammatory effect. If you choose flaxseed oil as the primary source of omega 3, then it is essential that you have adequate levels of vitamin B6, magnesium and zinc, as these nutrients are necessary to convert the fat in the flaxseed oil into its anti-inflammatory form. If you are not vegetarian I would recommend fish body oil to better achieve the desired effects on your pains and swellings.

What about cod liver oil?

Cod liver oil has been traditionally used for many years. People often recall taking a spoonful of cod liver oil each morning before school, given to them by their health-conscious parents. This habit has died out nowadays, but the benefits of this kind of routine intake should not be disregarded. Cod liver oil can be a very useful supplement, but in most cases of arthritis, one tends to gain a better result from using the oil from the body of the fish rather than the liver. The reason for this is that cod liver oil contains vitamins A and D as well as the active ingredient, omega 3. These vitamins are generally very beneficial to the body, but care needs to be exercised when consuming high levels of individual vitamins; when taken in excess they will be stored in the body and potentially cause imbalances. If you obtain a sufficient level of omega 3 from the cod liver oil, therefore, it is likely that the concurrent dose of vitamins A and D will be too much for you. There are of course exceptions: when a high level of Vitamin A or D is required, cod liver oil may be the right choice.

Purity and contamination issues of essential fat supplements

As fish oil products are obviously sourced from fish, the contaminants present in the oceans and other waters from which fish are obtained must be filtered out somehow. Substances that may be harmful to us, such as mercury and dioxins, creep into our food chain via their accumulation within the bodies of fish that reside in polluted waters. There are various methods of removing them to ensure that the end product is completely free from anything potentially harmful. Product choice and selection is crucial if you are to avoid ending up with a poorly purified product containing residues of these toxins, all of which have well-documented negative health effects.

Many health supplements are sourced from tuna. Being a larger predatory fish, tuna is often found to contain high levels of toxins as it accumulates not only those from the seas but also those of the fish it has eaten over its lifetime. Provided an extensive purification process is undergone, the end product should be absolutely fine; however, this might be where cheaper supplements fall short.

Salmon is another great source of omega 3 fish oil products. If obtained from the cleaner seas off Alaska or Norway, for example – waters that are still relatively unpolluted – this fish (and any supplements derived from it) is certainly a safer option to eat than tuna, especially if it is marked as 'wild' salmon.

Liquid or capsule supplements?

I tend to recommend the liquid 'off the spoon' way of taking fish oils as the most effective. You can take in a much higher dose relatively easily compared to taking the same dose in capsules. If taken with food for better absorption, more of the anti-inflammatory substance is available to your body from a teaspoon than within a capsule. You would need to take more than one capsule to match the teaspoon dose. Consider your digestive system, which has to break open the capsules to absorb their contents. As many people with arthritis are on a lot of medication already, it could be argued that yet another capsule or tablet may not be absorbed as well as it should be. Personal preference may dictate the option you choose: some people cannot tolerate the taste or texture of the oil and would rather have it encapsulated, in which case a higher potency product will probably be necessary.

These issues may all seem very confusing. How are you supposed to pick a good product off the shelves with all this in mind? Product leaflets from the manufacturer can be very useful and are normally available in the health shop that sells the product. These often mention the purification method used and contain the claims that the toxins have been filtered out to well below the minimum safe levels. If the leaflet doesn't mention this, then it is quite likely that it is a poor product. Staff in health food shops, particularly independent stores, should know this sort of information and will hopefully be of great assistance in making the choice.

Research on essential fat supplements

A great deal of research has been carried out on the use of fish oils in the treatment of diseases such as arthritis. It is now fairly well accepted that the use of these oils is very beneficial as part of a treatment for pain and inflammation. For example, clinical trials have found anti-inflammatory benefits of omega 3 fatty acids while experiments have shown that omega 3 helps prevent the breakdown of cartilage by enzymes.[13] They are thought to act by inhibiting the COX-2 enzymes and other inflammatory mediators. (An example of a pharmaceutical COX-2 inhibitor is celebrex/celecoxib.)

Omega 3 supplements consistently demonstrate an improvement in symptoms and also a reduction in the use of NSAIDs, the common non-steroidal anti-inflammatory drugs often prescribed for arthritis.[14] In *Arthritis and Rheumatism*, it was found that some patients who take fish oils can stop taking their NSAIDs without experiencing a flare-up of their condition.[15]

Dosage information

Fish oil: EPA 750–2,000 mg, DHA 500–1,500 mg per daily intake. This dose applies to both liquid products and capsules. Vitamin E or rosemary oil may be added within the formulation to help protect the freshness of the oil. If it is not included, ensure that you take some vitamin E within a multinutrient formula or on its own.

Flaxseed oil: For liquid flaxseed oil, preferably organic, take 1–2 teaspoons each day and also add to foods, or sprinkle on to salads and vegetables. Do not heat this oil.

Flaxseed oil capsules: 1,000–3,000 mg per daily intake. About 50 to 60 per cent of the oil will provide omega 3 while the remaining portion provides omega 6 and 9 also.

Cautions

If you are taking warfarin or a blood thinning medicine, please consult your doctor before taking fish oils.

Discontinue fish oil two weeks before a surgical procedure.

Glossary of terms

Omega 3 fatty acid   A beneficial type of fat, known to have anti-inflammatory properties. The omega 3 term describes its chemical structure as compared with other fats, for example omega 6.

EPA (eicosapentanoic acid)   A polyunsaturated omega 3 fatty acid, found predominantly in oily fish.

DHA (docosohexanoic acid) A polyunsaturated omega 3 fatty acid. DHA is a vital structural part of our brain and eyes. DHA can be produced from EPA or obtained from the diet or fish oil supplements.

Essential fatty acid Those fats that the human body requires for its biological functions but cannot synthesize itself. These fats must be obtained through dietary means.

Trans fat Not an essential fat, trans fats have no known benefit to human health. These types of fats are associated with an increased risk of heart disease and potentially many other health problems. There are some naturally occurring trans fats in animal products and dairy foods; however, most of the damaging fats come from processed foods and techniques such as deep fat frying.

Saturated fat These should be reduced in the diet of those with arthritis as an excess can cause greater levels of inflammation. They are also thought to contribute to cardiovascular disease. Saturated fats are found in animal products such as butter, cream, cheese and fatty meats. Chocolate and processed foods tend to be a source of this detrimental fat.

Polyunsaturated fat Found mainly within nuts and seeds, fish, algae, leafy green vegetables. Omega 3 is classed as a polyunsaturated fat. This group of fats is considered the most beneficial in treating arthritis.

Monounsaturated fat Olive oil is a good source of monounsaturated fat along with avocados, nuts, grapeseed oil, groundnut oil and sesame oil.

Option 5: Herbal solutions

We are currently in the process of real change regarding the availability of herbal medicines to the public. In Europe, the United Kingdom and the USA many restrictions have been placed on what consumers are able to purchase from health stores. Many herbs will need to be prescribed by a medical herbalist and those that are freely available to purchase will need to carry a medicinal licence once their effects have been scientifically proven and accepted.

This is an extremely costly process, and therefore many herbs have simply been taken off the shelves for the time being as many of the manufacturers cannot keep up with the regulation. As it is such a time of change, it is hard to predict what the future availability of good quality herbal treatments will be.

The aim of this book is to impart plenty of information for people with arthritis, enabling them to choose their own comprehensive natural treatment. I will therefore discuss only the more popular, well-known herbal pain relievers that are likely to remain available.

As I outlined in the previous section, there are several nutritional products available that can help relieve the pain and inflammation of arthritis. This means that you don't have to rely solely on the herbal varieties to ensure a successful recovery. The licensing issue may simply make the decision easier, as there is now less choice than there has been in recent years.

Dietary herbs can still be easily incorporated and most of the commonly grown kitchen herbs can be very beneficial to overall health. They are easy to grow in gardens or on kitchen window sills and a handful can be added to most dishes for extra flavour and nutritional benefit. Examples of these culinary herbs include coriander, parsley, mint and cumin.

Ginger and turmeric, described fully in this section, can be used in their food forms, regardless of their availability as a supplement. Of course, the supplement version will normally be a lot stronger, more concentrated and have faster effects, but the food version can be easily incorporated several times weekly into a normal diet, which will still allow you to gain its broader benefits.

Ginger

A well-known herbal medicine, ginger (*Zingiber officinale*) has been used for many thousands of years. The root is the part commonly used in herbal preparations and for cooking.

In Ayurvedic (traditional Indian) medicine, ginger is used to treat many types of health concerns as well as for its effects on pain and inflammation. It prevents gas within the digestive tract, prevents spasms of the stomach or intestine, relieves nausea, heartburn and indigestion, clears the lungs of mucus, stimulates circulation and appetite, and drains excess fluid from the body, i.e. it acts as a diuretic.

These beneficial effects of ginger illustrate the many positive effects on total body health that may be achieved when taking natural treatments. It might help you to choose whether ginger is the right option for your arthritis if you also have poor circulation and inadequate digestion, for example.

The following scientific research studies have investigated ginger as a pain-relieving, anti-inflammatory treatment:

- A study in 2011 found that ginger was 'remarkably effective for the treatment of acute gout arthritis'.[16]
- In 2009, a comparison of a ginger product with the rheumatoid arthritis medication methotrexate showed the ginger product was equally effective for the treatment of rheumatoid arthritis due to its anti-inflammatory effects.[17]
- When 261 osteoarthritis patients were given a ginger extract for six weeks, it was observed to have a significant effect in reducing symptoms in osteoarthritis of the knee. It was found to be safe, with only a mild gastrointestinal adverse effect in some people.[18]
- Tests have shown ginger to reduce swelling and inhibit the inflammatory mediators cyclooxygenase (COX) and lipooxygenase (LOX) and also leukotriene synthesis. These substances are often targeted by pharmaceutical medications to control pain and inflammation.[19]
- A study of the effects of ginger on osteoarthritis, rheumatoid arthritis and those with muscle discomfort found that 75 per cent of all patients studied saw improvements in swelling and pain. Interestingly, all the people with muscle discomfort experienced relief.[20]

Cautions

Existing gastrointestinal complaints such as stomach ulcers or hiatus hernia may be aggravated by ginger – discontinue use if this is the case.

Those with gallstones or bile duct obstruction should seek professional advice.

Ginger may have anticoagulant effects. You should therefore also seek professional advice if you are taking a blood-thinning medication such as warfarin, or aspirin.

Turmeric

A close relative of ginger, turmeric (*Curcuma longa*) has long been used in Indian medicine as a powerful anti-inflammatory. Its active constituent, curcumin, appears to be much safer than using a traditional prescribed medicine to achieve a similar outcome.

In addition to its anti-inflammatory and pain-relieving effects, extract of curcumin has been shown to prevent the breakdown of joint components including hyaluronic acid and collagen.[21]

I mentioned earlier the use of antioxidants in helping to relieve the symptoms of arthritis and also in preventing further damage from occurring. Turmeric exerts very powerful antioxidant effects in addition to its well-known anti-inflammatory properties. As an antioxidant, turmeric is able to neutralize free radicals, particularly those responsible for painful joint inflammation and subsequent damage.

Turmeric works better if taken with black pepper. Piperine, found within black pepper, enhances its uptake into the bloodstream. Earlier I mentioned that the action of natural remedies is often improved by co-factors that in some way to help the body either absorb or utilize the active ingredient. Piperine is one of these co-factors as it helps build even further on the beneficial effects of curcumin.

If you take it in your diet, use turmeric alongside black pepper within the same dish. Buy organic turmeric if possible as this will be free from irradiation, a process commonly applied to herbs that end up on supermarket shelves. Curry powders tend to contain only a small amount of turmeric, so it is best to buy the single spice on its own. It can be added to scrambled eggs, vegetables, onions and casseroles, or even added to juices.

Cautions

Those with gallstones or bile duct obstruction should seek professional advice.

Existing gastrointestinal complaints such as gastroesophageal reflux disease, stomach ulcers or hiatus hernia may be aggravated by curcumin – discontinue use if this is the case.

Curcumin may have anticoagulant effects, therefore seek professional advice if you are taking a blood-thinning medication such as warfarin or aspirin.

Curcumin is best absorbed when taken with meals.

Boswellia

Boswellic acids are the active constituents of boswellia (*Boswellia serrata*), also known as frankincense. These compounds are thought to act by inhibiting the body's process of inflammation in a similar way to how prescribed anti-inflammatory drugs work for arthritis.

Many research studies have found boswellia to possess activity against arthritis. One of these studies followed 260 patients with rheumatoid arthritis and it was found that 50 to 60 per cent of those who took boswellia experienced a significant reduction in joint pain, swelling and morning stiffness.[22] Their general health and well-being also improved while they were taking this herb.

It appears to be a very safe way of reducing the pain and inflammation of the condition. In a research study on boswellia for arthritis, no significant side effects or toxicity were found, unlike most prescribed anti-inflammatory medications.[23]

Devil's claw

Devil's claw (*Harpagophytum procumbens*) has anti-inflammatory and pain-relieving properties and is a popular choice for those with both osteoarthritis and rheumatoid arthritis. Its effectiveness has been likened to non-steroidal anti-inflammatory drugs such as ibuprofen and also the COX-2 inhibitors such as celecoxib, but without the risk of side effects that goes with these prescribed medications.

To quote the research, devil's claw is 'an effective and well-tolerated serious treatment option for mild to moderate degenerative rheumatic disorders providing improved quality of life'.[24]

Cautions

Devil's claw has an effect on stomach acid, so it is not advised for people with gastritis, heartburn, ulcers or any other form of excess acid within the digestive system.

Those with gallstones should seek professional advice before taking devil's claw.

General note on herbal solutions for pain and inflammation

These substances can be extremely useful for all types of arthritis. However, they must not be used alone and must be combined with treatments included in Categories 1 and 2 to achieve proper recovery. Some people find they gain such great relief by using the herbal treatments that they neglect the underlying cause of their arthritis, as their symptoms are well under control. It is brilliant if you can control your symptoms using herbal alternatives to prescribed painkillers and anti-inflammatories, but make sure that you use them correctly and in conjunction with the rest of the programme.

6

Sample treatment plans

This chapter includes some sample plans that will help you envisage the sort of treatment programme you might choose to undertake. Each of the five plans is different, being designed to accommodate varying levels of illness, mobility and other factors.

Each plan provides suggestions only and should be taken as a general guide rather than an exact prescription. The main message is to take aspects from each of the three categories of treatment to give yourself the best chance of success.

Organizations listed in the Useful addresses section can give you further help and guidance, and supply personalized treatment plans.

Treatment plan 1

This plan will suit the following:

- those with the physical ability to prepare and cook food;
- those who can safely climb in and out of the bath;
- those with a milder form of arthritis, e.g. those who are still able to work or carry out normal daily activities.

The plan consists of the following six elements:

1 *An alkaline diet* Those with milder arthritis can incorporate many more of the dietary recommendations than those whose arthritis inhibits their abilities in the kitchen. Try to follow these guidelines:
   - Include a plentiful quantity of steamed vegetables. Vary the type and ideally buy a seasonal vegetable box to ensure a broad variety of nutrients from the different vegetables that each season provides. Use a variety of colours of vegetables, remembering to avoid tomatoes.

- Oily fish such as mackerel or sardines should be eaten at least twice a week, if not more. This will provide the essential fatty acids needed to combat the inflammation in your joints.
- White fish can be eaten, providing a good protein source, as can chicken, turkey and various legume protein sources such as lentils and beans.
- Add herbs and spices to your foods, including ginger and turmeric for their anti-inflammatory activity and parsley, basil, mint and coriander to provide antioxidants and chlorophyll.
- Have a balanced mix of raw, uncooked foods (such as salad vegetables) and cooked/steamed foods.
- Drinks include green tea, mint tea, nettle tea, fresh ginger root tea and water.

2 *Cider vinegar and Epsom salts* These naturopathic remedies should be easy to incorporate into a routine. They offer powerful benefits for all types of arthritis and will help ensure a good night's sleep, while providing the minerals for recovery. If you work all day, you can make up your cider vinegar drinks in the morning and take them with you. For a day's intake, use a pint of water and add 3 dessertspoonfuls cider vinegar and 3 teaspoons honey unless diabetic. The baths should easily fit into your routine – remember, you only need to soak for 10 to 15 minutes to get the benefits.

3 *Molasses* – 1–3 teaspoons daily. If you are constipated, use the maximum dose of 3 teaspoons at intervals throughout the day, on an empty stomach.

4 *Multinutrient formula* Your diet will provide many nutrients. However, the potency of a high quality multinutrient formula will enable a faster recovery. When you have arthritis, even mildly, it is very difficult to meet the high demands of your body for nutrients to facilitate the repair of joints while meeting antioxidant requirements.

5 *Protein supplement* Even though the diet provides substantial amounts of protein, this supplement is still needed to ensure repair of the affected joints.

6 *Digestive enzymes* Additional pain relief can be obtained by using these on an empty stomach. For mild forms of arthritis, this extra pain relief may not be necessary. It is likely to be useful as and when needed, i.e. during a flare-up, rather than continuously.

Treatment plan 2

This plan is ideally suited for:

- those unable to get in and out of the bath;
- those with limited mobility or who are housebound;
- those unable to cook or prepare food without assistance.

It consists of the following eight elements:

1 *Multinutrient formula* As the diet is poor, coupled with severe arthritis, the body's requirements for nutrients in this case are extremely high. To meet such high demands, it is necessary to take a high potency multinutrient formula.
2 *Green supplement* To provide condensed nutrition and alkalize the body in as easy a form as possible.
3 *Cider vinegar* To alkalize the body, large batches may be made in advance by a carer, for example, and left unrefrigerated within reach.
4 *Glucosamine and chondroitin* When you have extremely limited joint movement, these supplements can be very beneficial.
5 *Protein powder* Use this in order to improve your dietary intake of protein, ideally in addition to meals rather than as a replacement for them. Take twice daily if the diet is poor to ensure adequate repair nutrients for the joints.
6 *DLPA* Those who are bed bound or have equally limited mobility bear the constant everyday pain of arthritis. DLPA can provide lasting, effective relief from the pain. In such cases, pain may still be felt but it should be easier to cope with.
7 *Enzymes* In addition to their anti-inflammatory and pain-relieving effects, enzyme products help the circulation, especially when there is significant lack of movement. This should help to prevent blood clots and other circulatory complications of being bed bound.
8 *Magnesium spray or gel* Apply to the painful areas as often as needed. The skin may initially tingle when the spray or gel is applied.

This may seem like a lot to take on. Remember to start slowly and introduce the supplements gradually, as you feel able. You may not need all of the above treatments and will hopefully find some to try that you feel suit your own situation. Three different types of natural pain relief are mentioned in this programme. One of these may suffice, but if your pain is severe and constant you may need to try adding one of the other options. As you start to feel better and it becomes easier for you to move around, you can start to think about preparing food and introducing the dietary recommendations to alkalize your body even further. At this stage, you may find you can leave off the green supplement and reduce the servings of protein powder to one each day. As the pain becomes easier still to cope with, perhaps next you could leave off the enzymes and rely on DLPA alone to provide the pain relief. At this time, it may be possible to introduce a foot bath of Epsom salts, eventually progressing to a full body soak when you find it easier and safer to get in and out of the bath.

Treatment plan 3

This plan is suited to the following people:

- those who have not only arthritis but also some other condition such as anaemia, cardiovascular disease, depression or thyroid dysfunction (both overactive and underactive);
- those with multiple and complex health issues, perhaps entailing high levels of medication.

1 *Greens*   Potent alkalizing of the body using concentrated greens will have a balancing effect on the entire body. Green supplements may help the correction of anaemia by nourishing the blood cells. Some people may find their other conditions improve as time goes on.
2 *Alkaline diet*   Removing the acid foods from your diet benefits many aspects of your health, reducing inflammation and normalising the immune system.
3 *Epsom salts*   The lack of energy associated with any of the above health conditions may be alleviated by Epsom salts baths.
4 *Cider vinegar and honey drinks*   The multitude of benefits attributed to cider vinegar relate to all the conditions mentioned. It may reduce blood pressure and cholesterol level via its high potassium content and ability to detoxify the blood.
5 *Multinutrient formula*   Those with multiple and/or complex health issues are very likely to have vitamin and mineral deficiencies. A good formulation will start to correct these deficiencies, enabling the rest of the treatment to work properly.
6 *Enzymes*   Can be safely taken alongside medication. While helping relieve the pain of arthritis, enzymes improve the health of the cardiovascular system by clearing arterial deposits, ensuring good blood flow and reducing inflammation.

7 *Omega 3* Fish oil provides additional benefits for the cardiovascular system and reducing inflammation anywhere in the body. Use with caution if taking anti-coagulant medication such as warfarin.

There is even more emphasis in this programme on alkalizing the body. When you have a multitude of complex health problems and different conditions, it indicates a long-standing imbalance of the acid/alkaline levels in your body. In these cases, progress is likely to be better if the programme is focused on restoring this crucial balance.

Treatment plan 4

This plan is suitable for those who cannot swallow tablets or capsules. Many people struggle to swallow pills of any description without difficulty. This may be due to disease of or an obstruction of the throat or oesophagus; some simply fear tablets getting stuck. The plan consists of the following elements:

1 *High quality liquid multinutrient formula* Follow the same advice as given earlier with regard to dosage;
or
Sublingual multinutrient formula Sublingual literally means 'under the tongue'. A good way to take supplements if you have some trouble swallowing is to have a sublingual powder that you place underneath your tongue, where it will dissolve straight into the veins situated there. The nutrient passes straight into your bloodstream and is very effective at raising levels of that essential substance when otherwise supplementation may not be effective. This is also useful if you have digestive difficulties and consequently experience problems in absorbing nutrients.

2 *Liquid omega 3 from fish oil.*

3 *Epsom salts baths* The magnesium and sulphur are both absorbed through the skin into your body where they are needed. It is a very effective way of obtaining these two nutrients, more so than taking an oral supplement. If you are unable to get in or out of the bath, magnesium is available as a liquid, powder or magnesium oil spray, or as homeopathic tissue salts that dissolve on your tongue.

4 *Liquid ginger* Available as a natural anti-inflammatory option, or grate fresh root ginger into hot water.

5 *Cider vinegar* If you have disease of the oesophagus or upper digestive tract, start slowly with cider vinegar. For example, start with only

1 teaspoon (5 ml) well diluted in 300 ml of water. Add honey (if you are not diabetic), as the healing properties of this may help to calm inflammation within the digestive tract.
6 *Protein powder*   This can be sprinkled on to food or dissolved into a drink.

You can see there are many options for those who cannot swallow tablets, so this difficulty shouldn't limit your improvement in any way.

Treatment plan 5

This plan is suited to those with extremely limited finances.

Financial difficulties are very common among people with arthritis. This may be due to the loss of income from being unable to work or possibly due to age and receiving only a small pension. These people still need help and there are ways to achieve a successful outcome, despite the lack of funds.

Acupuncture is now available free of charge on the National Health Service and can help you improve your pain and energy balance. However, there is generally no funding available for nutritional supplements. You may be entitled to prescribed supplements from your GP. These may not be ideal in terms of what they provide but should still offer some benefit. Possible options include various vitamins and minerals, omega 3 products and vitamin B12 injections. This route may be worth investigating, but bear in mind that the supplements may be of lower quality than those available to buy independently.

You may wish to seek advice from a nutritional therapist who can discuss with you your financial restrictions and recommend exactly what you need. This ensures you spend your money as productively as possible rather than buying several cheap supplements, which is often a false economy. Emphasis will be put on the actions you can take to improve in your diet rather than buying supplements.

1 *Maximize the use of your food* in the following ways:
   • Never throw away vegetables or leave them sitting in the fridge. Make a soup or casserole out of them using your own stock (see below), as most vegetable flavours will combine fairly well.
   • Make your own stock by following the directions given in Chapter 4 (see p. 50). Ask your local butcher for his leftover chicken bones or lamb bones; often they are given away.
   • Use apple peelings, washed, steeped in boiling water and drink as tea.

- Grate fresh root ginger into hot water and take as a drink for pain relief.
- Once you have cooked vegetables, retain the water and drink it. It will be full of nutrients.
- Use vegetarian sources of protein. Foods such as lentils and beans are far cheaper to buy than meat.
- Make large batches of meals to stretch the ingredients as far as possible. Freeze these and reheat in the oven when needed.
- Do not use a microwave as it destroys nutrients.

2 *Drink diluted cider vinegar* This is an absolute must for those with limited financial resources.

3 *Sublingual multinutrient formulas* These tend to be cheaper as their production cost is lower. They are powders, so you can adjust the dose you take as much as you like or can afford. For example, if a month's supply costs £10, you could take a quarter of the dose and make your pot of powdered nutrients last for four months. This takes the cost down to £2.50 for each month's worth. It will not act so quickly but it is better than taking nothing or a cheap, poor quality supplement.

4 *Flaxseed oil* Use as a source of omega 3 and drizzle on to salads and meals. Do not heat. This may provide some reduction in inflammation but is not as potent as taking a fish oil or concentrated flaxseed supplement.

It is always better to do something rather than nothing at all. All your efforts will help you enormously in many aspects of your health. If some months you can afford a little extra, spend it on some Epsom salts for your bath or one of the multinutrient formulas.

Family members or good friends will see that you are trying as hard as you can to make yourself better and will be willing to help out in some way, whether by providing food or by offering a little financial support. They will want to see you well again as soon as possible. If help is offered, don't be afraid to take it!

Look closely at your weekly shop. Are you spending money on cordials, ready-prepared foods, biscuits or snacks, alcohol, branded toiletries or cleaning products? There may be some areas of your lifestyle where you can save money so that it is available to spend on fresh food and supplements instead. Your health is the most important aspect of your life. It is worth making sacrifices for wherever you possibly can.

7

Putting it all together

This chapter summarizes all the things you need to consider when planning your steps to recovery.

Often people prefer to start with small steps, gradually adapting to the changes involved. The foundation of all nutritional programmes to conquer arthritis should begin with the following as a bare minimum. This basic grounding can then be built upon to suit your individual circumstances:

1 Ensure vitamin and mineral sufficiency.
2 Begin an alkalizing technique from Category 1 such as drinking cider vinegar or bathing in Epsom salts (see Chapter 3).
3 Start addressing your diet by gradually removing the more acid foods and eating more of the alkalizing foods.

Please note: this is a good starting point, but you will need to add to it gradually by incorporating other elements from Categories 2 and 3 in order to achieve the desired results of eliminating the symptoms of arthritis (see Chapters 4 and 5).

The first step I would recommend when starting to put together a treatment plan from the items discussed in previous chapters is to ensure an adequate intake of valuable vitamins and minerals, first and foremost through the diet and then in supplement form via multinutrient combination products, as I described earlier. A lack of vitamins and minerals will impair the body's ability to repair itself, so it is crucially important that this is addressed before choosing the remaining aspects of the programme. Use the information in Chapter 4, on joint repair nutrients, to make a good choice of product.

You might want to introduce this plan in small, manageable stages rather than launch into too many changes at once. This is perfectly acceptable. You can do the above basics for four to six weeks or so and let your body gradually adapt. Products can then be added to the programme one by one while making your diet increasingly alkaline over time.

It is sensible to go about changes slowly, all the while letting your body system accommodate them. This time can be used to ensure that no inhibiting problems arise. One common example of such a problem is constipation. If you have a history of bowel trouble, it is important to address this in the initial stages of the programme. If adequate elimination is not carried out via the bowels, then your body will not be able to get rid of the acid residues that are causing the arthritis. The natural choice for a person with constipation would be molasses from Category 1, as this acts as a mild laxative when taken on an empty stomach.

The same applies to other ongoing health problems. By viewing the body as a whole system, it becomes clearer how each isolated problem is actually part of the arthritis, or has contributed to its onset in some way. All the problems and symptoms present initially should improve from this natural approach as it normalizes your body processes.

The only way to successful recovery is through building a comprehensive programme. Such changes may feel very daunting at first, particularly when you are feeling unwell or are housebound by your arthritis. If it all seems too much, then break it down in the above way and gradually add in more components from each of the categories as time goes on and you start to feel up to it. It will not be a problem to start really slowly and persevere through each stage in your own time.

Ten points to remember when planning your treatment programme

Allow time

If you use the approach I have outlined in this book, you are likely to notice improvements in your general health first of all. However, it may take several weeks before you are aware of any noticeable improvements in your arthritis. And it is likely to take you several months or even a few years to achieve a *complete* recovery. The rule of thumb for naturopathic healing is to allow one month of recovery for every year the condition has been present to see a true reversal of such a chronic condition. For example, if your joint pains began 15 years ago, you might anticipate it will be necessary to undertake a 15-month treatment programme before recovery. Sometimes it is quicker than this but, for whatever reason, it may also be slower – everyone is different. Having said that, this rule of thumb helps – if you know what to expect in terms of what progress you make, your compliance and motivation will be better.

Commit wholeheartedly

Once the settling-in period has passed, all three categories of the programme should be adhered to consistently. I have seen many occasions when people attempt such a programme half-heartedly only to be
extremely disappointed when it takes a long time to see results. It may
feel like a huge burden at the time but, even for slow recovery, it is a very
short period considering how long most people put up with some sort
of joint pain before really dealing with it. Try to be as compliant as you
are able, but know that if you slip up and forget what you are meant to
be doing, simply draw a line under it and start again. Look forward at
all times and forget the past. If you frequently slip up it will take much
longer to get there, but you will still recover if you put your mind to it.

Expect flare-ups of pain

Flare-ups are likely to occur as part of the normal course of treatment.
The first flare-up often occurs within the first few weeks of starting complete treatment. It is due to the fact that deep-rooted acidity is being
drawn out and is mobilizing around the body. This is beneficial as part
of the healing process, but it can be very painful, and your arthritis may
seem to feel worse at this point, or even more widespread. However,
it does pass, usually relatively quickly (perhaps a few days or within a
couple of weeks), and afterwards you should feel much better. It is particularly important at this stage not to lose faith but to keep going with
your programme as it is clearing the acid. Drink plenty of fluids and
ensure your bowels are opening daily.

Allow yourself adequate rest

Rest, relaxation and sleep provide the ideal opportunity for your body
to heal. Poor sleep can be a problem due to pain or discomfort. This
should gradually restore itself as time goes on, but focus should be given
to rest times during the day. Often, people think of resting as laziness.
However, it is a crucial part of recovery and should be taken seriously.
Short naps in the daytime are perfectly acceptable if that is what your
body is telling you it needs.

Keep as active as your body allows

As your joints need to be used in order to enable them to heal and
work effectively again, it is advisable to take gentle exercise when you

are capable of it. Using a frame to improve your stability might help if your confidence is low and you should try each day to get on your feet. Levels of exercise and activity vary hugely, dependent on the severity of the arthritis. Some people might not even be able to get out of bed without assistance at first and the initial goal for these people might be simply to walk to the bathroom unaided. Others, despite arthritis, overdo exercise. Excessive running or excessive cycling, for example, is not advised. Keep all exercise gentle.

Keep a record of your symptoms

Start keeping a record of all your symptoms at the beginning of the programme. Make a note of everything you feel is abnormal within your body, e.g. feeling tired all the time, high blood pressure, irritable bowel syndrome, eczema/skin complaints, frequent headaches, depression, anxiety, muscle aches, etc. This list might be frighteningly long at the outset, but use it to monitor how much better you are at the end of each month. It will help motivate you to keep persevering with the programme.

Think positively and consider your future

Keep your 'post-arthritis' life in mind frequently. Thinking about and visualizing a life of free mobility and without pain will help you to achieve that life. You will no longer have the limitations that are holding you back now. A positive state of mind not only helps you to get through each day, but also might lead to a faster recovery. It will certainly help to keep you on track through difficult times.

Use all the aids available

There is no shame in using a stick or frame for a period of time, no matter what age you are. Know that you will soon be able to throw it away. These aids will make your life easier and safer from day to day while you are undergoing this recovery programme. Many companies supply arthritic aids for the household, to assist mobility, dressing, driving, etc. Use whatever is available.

Acknowledge the stress in your life

Identifying the source of stress is the first step to dealing with that stress. This is important, as it has a direct impact on your body's ability to heal. Often, chronic stress can be dealt with nutritionally in order to help you cope better. It is not easy to eradicate stresses from your life and it may well be impossible without drastic changes to your situation; if that is the case, the best way to deal with it is to focus on supporting your body through it rather than trying to get rid of the stress itself.

If in doubt, ask for help

Since my grandmother, Margaret Hills, established our clinic in the early 1980s, we have specialized in the natural treatment of arthritis and in offering support to those going through a recovery programme. We offer individualized, tailored programmes and guidance to help you achieve your goals. We have personal experience of the condition and can strongly empathize with each individual situation. To help you keep positive, we can put you in touch with other people with arthritis for support. This might be someone your own age or with a similar diagnosis, or someone living in your area, so you could potentially meet. This is an entirely optional scheme offered only to those registered with us.

How to choose a good quality supplement

The *Journal of the American Medical Association* declared in 2002 that 'suboptimal intake of some vitamins, above levels causing classic vitamin deficiency, is a risk factor for chronic diseases and common in the general population'.[1] The report also commented that most people's diets do not provide the nutrient requirements; therefore supplementation is becoming necessary. Due to the worldwide depletion of soil quality, food and therefore people are deficient in a wide array of nutrients. Even organic soils contain inadequate quantities of what we need.

There are many food supplements of vitamins and minerals on the market, their effectiveness ranging from excellent to really quite poor. This section is designed to help provide some clarity on what to look for when you are in a health food shop.

The price of supplements and false economies

The cost of supplements might be an issue, particularly when you are purchasing a full programme rather than just one product, so this has to be balanced out with effectiveness. Cheap supplements, however, are often a false economy. In most cases, it will be more cost effective to buy better quality products, although these are likely to be more expensive, but then to take less than the recommended dose – this will make the pot last longer. This way you will be getting the benefit of good quality nutrients, although it may take longer to see the desired improvement.

Beware of special offers on already cheap supplements. Some stores offer almost permanent discounts on their products. Good quality does cost money and if these supplements have a very low retail value then it is very likely that low quality ingredients are used in the manufacturing process. This isn't always the case, as some genuine incentives may be available; however, don't be led too easily by tempting offers.

Reputable companies will often reject a raw ingredient for quality reasons if it doesn't meet their minimum requirements for purity, potency or contamination. Cheaper ingredients may fall short of these quality requirements and are often used by manufacturers who have less stringent quality limits. For example, chemical solvents can be used in the extraction of phytonutrients from herbs. Let us next take a look at specific types of supplements to help you choose the right product.

Mineral supplements

Magnesium, calcium and zinc are all examples of minerals found in supplement form. The body cannot metabolize them as individual elements; they have to be transported into the blood. The type of transporter is very important as some are far more effective than others. For example, you may read on the label 'Magnesium Citrate' when citrate is the carrier of magnesium.

Citrate and malate forms are very good. These carriers have well-researched metabolic functions within the body so once it has delivered the mineral into the body, the carrier then has a useful job to perform.

Amino acid chelates tend to be advantageous transporters.

Carbonate and sulphate forms are very common but are not well absorbed by the body and most of the supplement may be wasted. However, diluted cider vinegar, for example, helps improve the breakdown of the supplement and its subsequent absorption into the body.

Oxide forms have poor uptake by the body and can often be irritating to the digestive tract.

Another well-recommended type of supplement is 'food state'. These types are manufactured in a way that replicates a mineral in a food form so it is easier for the body to recognize and use it. Food state products are the closest you can get to the natural state of the original nutrient in a supplement form. Absorption of these food forms of supplements tends to be very good and, as a result, they normally provide a lower dose than a standard supplement. Some suppliers claim that they are about four times stronger than the label dose suggests if a like-for-like comparison is made. For example, to obtain the equivalent of 400 mg of magnesium from a standard form, one would take 100 mg of a food state version.

Unwanted additional ingredients

Check the label for inactive ingredients. Using magnesium as an example, Magnesium itself is the 'active' ingredient. All others listed are normally 'inactive'; they are present purely as a base or tabletting/encapsulation ingredient used in the manufacturing process.

Reputable companies use minimal amounts of inactive ingredients, only those essential to create the finished product. If the list is long, some of these ingredients may not be necessary.

Artificial sweeteners are used in some poor quality products, as are other unnecessary ingredients such as artificial flavourings, excessive filling agents and coatings. Avoid these if possible and look for a purer product.

Sweeteners

Some products, particularly protein powders, may be sweetened to make them more palatable. However, there are a few natural sweeteners that are quite safe to include. These are xylitol (the crystallized form of sweet sap from the birch tree), agave (syrup from the leaves of this Mediterranean plant) and fructose (fruit sugar) in small amounts.

Sweeteners to avoid include aspartame, acesulfame K, saccharin and high fructose corn syrup, as these may be detrimental to your health.

Soya protein

Most of the world's soya products are now genetically modified (GM). Always check that your supplement has 'non-GM' on the label as this is the only version I would recommend you use.

Amount or dose per capsule or per daily intake?

This is one of the major sources of confusion for people buying supplements. Not only are the words difficult to read as there is so much information packed on to the label, but it can be hard to see how much you will be taking each day. For example, on a tub of fish oil, it may state 'high potency fish oil 1,000 mg'. This is misleading, as you might think that you are taking a sufficient amount when in fact the amounts of the beneficial elements, EPA and DHA, are actually only 160 mg and 100 mg respectively. This often catches people out, so take care to read the list of active ingredients on the label and see how much of those you are getting.

Combination supplements

You may find that certain nutrients are grouped together to deliver the correct combination for your problems. For example, a specialist combination may include glucosamine sulphate, chondroitin sulphate, quercetin, MSM, ginger and rosehips. This combination would be targeted at people with arthritis as a broad-spectrum joint support formula. Some of these products can be quite a good way of obtaining a variety of nutrients without having to take too many tablets or capsules. It can also be quite cost effective to purchase these types of combinations. On the other hand, if you need just one ingredient specifically to deal with an existing deficiency of that nutrient, you will have to choose a single product that contains only that nutrient, otherwise the dose may be too low for you. Refer to the section in Chapter 4 regarding multinutrient combination formulas for further help.

8

Exercise and joint health

In addition to your diet and supplement programme, there are other aspects of treatment that require consideration. The exercise you choose to undertake can either help your arthritis or make it worse, so it is worth understanding how exercise plays a role in the health of your joints. Exercising safely is very important whether you have arthritis or not, as inappropriate exercise, too much or too little, can be detrimental to joints.

If you are able to, it is beneficial to utilize your joints on a daily basis. Utilizing your joints can mean many things, dependent on the level of exercise you are capable of. For example, utilizing a joint will involve compressing and decompressing it, possibly while it is bearing weight. Bending and straightening your knee or walking on it would be considered to be utilizing the joint.

Periods of total inactivity of the joints soon affect the joint structure itself. If the joint is not compressed, no nutrients are delivered into the joint spaces and removal of waste products from the joints is impaired. This is due to the fact that there is no direct blood supply to cartilage. Normally nutrients are delivered to an area in the body via the circulating blood, which subsequently removes toxic waste products; this system continues to operate as long as the heart is pumping. The joints, however, with no direct blood supply, must rely on their dynamic compressing ability to do this job. An unused cartilage can be affected after only ten days or so of inactivity.[1]

Having said that, it is important for people without an arthritic condition to maintain a reasonable level of physical activity. It may be that arthritis is brought on by other conditions that cause immobility and then prevent you from using your healthy joints, for example by a fracture that requires the joint to be kept stable in a cast, or an operation requiring bed rest in order to recover, which consequently leave you susceptible to the onset of osteoarthritis. More often than not, over-exercising is an issue in the onset of arthritis. Too much joint movement, if not adequately prepared for, can actually accelerate breakdown of the joint.

Many of us regularly go to the gym, where we constantly work our joints with a variety of exercises and activities. This can be very beneficial for our health, particularly our cardiovascular health. However, joint health is often neglected in this typical scenario until something goes wrong. Looking after your joints when exercising is of the utmost importance if you are to prevent damage.

The following are among the most common dangers of over-exercising:

- Over-compression of the joint (i.e. putting too much weight or impact on it for a repeated or prolonged time) can cause problems with the inner workings of the joint, after which things start to go wrong. The cartilage can degrade and leave the bones eventually exposed so that movements become more and more painful.
- An inadequate diet will not provide sufficient nutrients to continually repair the joints, so the joint structures decline faster than they can be repaired.
- Over-exercising produces free radicals, the body's enemy, which can damage tissues if not adequately mopped up by antioxidants that neutralize them.

Exercising can be extremely beneficial to your overall health and well-being. However, this is true only if you do not overstrain, have a varied, balanced diet, and take the right nutritional supplements if training hard.

Extreme caution should be taken when the joints are swollen, as normal movement of such joints can cause further damage due to the impaired circulation to the joint. In this case, more damage can be done by trying to exercise the joint than by resting it. The main things to remember about joint movement are:

- If it hurts, don't do it.
- Be very wary of joint manipulation, particularly when the person manipulating the joint (for example a chiropractor or physiotherapist) is not experienced in dealing with severe cases of arthritis. Forcing a joint to move when it is rigid or even locked can do a great deal of harm. Arthritic joints need to be treated with extreme care. Always err on the side of caution if you are not sure of the risk of a particular movement or exercise.

There is no single piece of advice I can give you regarding exercise other than to be extremely careful and do things gradually. There is enormous individual variation among people with arthritis; some cannot even contemplate the smallest movement, while others may have quite an active lifestyle. So the level of exercise each individual is able to carry out will vary hugely.

9

Troubleshooting

There are many factors affecting an individual's health that make it very difficult to accurately predict the outcome of treatment, whether for arthritis or any other condition. In this chapter I will explore some of the common reasons why a person may not respond well to the recommendations I have given you in this book so that they can be addressed. These are:

- digestive problems
- medication
- constant stress
- poor diet
- not absorbing supplements well
- sleeping difficulties
- lack of compliance.

Digestive problems

This is a common obstacle in natural treatment. There is a motto in natural medicine that states 'The gut is the root of all disease'. This means that if you have a condition of the digestive system it will significantly impact on the overall health of your body. It affects nutrient absorption, food digestion, energy production, immune function (via lack of healthy bacteria), the ability to fight incoming germs, blood sugar balance, and other functions crucial to health. If you have irritable bowel syndrome, or an inflammatory bowel disorder such as Crohn's disease or diverticulitis, this needs to be addressed as part of your arthritis recovery programme. It is a good idea to seek the advice of a well-qualified practitioner to achieve this, as there are many naturopathic ways to cope with and overcome such problems.

In addition, if there are problems within your digestive system, you may not be able to absorb a tablet or capsule supplement properly. You may need to take liquid supplements instead, or even in some cases a sublingual product that is dissolved under the tongue, bypassing the digestive tract entirely.

Medication

Pharmaceutical medication tends to have a suppressive action in the body. It inhibits pain, inhibits an overactive immune system, kills infection, reduces blood pressure and cholesterol; all of which may be necessary and even life-saving at some point. However, this suppression of symptoms on a long-term basis only makes it harder for you to listen to your body's signals for help. Medication never seems to look at the cause.

- Why is the blood pressure or cholesterol high?
- Why is the immune system attacking the body?
- Why is there constant pain?
- Why is someone susceptible to frequent infections?

Medication does not answer these questions, it only stops the symptoms that give rise to them. For long-term health it is far more beneficial to use dietary and nutritional means to normalize your health irregularities. Addressing the stress or lifestyle and dietary factors that may be affecting your health is far more of a permanent fix than taking tablets for the rest of your life.

One of my favourite sayings is 'Headaches are not caused by a paracetamol deficiency'. It illustrates the way that we tend to suppress our symptoms rather than tackle the underlying cause.

There may be a different way to combat a particular health issue. Many people come to me armed with their current prescription, which can commonly be two or three pages long. Often people don't even know why they are taking a particular medicine or whether it is still necessary.

A very common situation is the repeated use of antibiotics for minor infections, each course causing even more detriment to the body's natural defences than the last. Many people have a terrible flare-up of their arthritis after a course of antibiotics as this tends to aggravate the pain. It is not to say the antibiotics weren't necessary but perhaps the necessity for their use should be questioned more often. We should focus instead on building up the natural resistance of the immune system.

If you are on medication, and are struggling with your arthritis among other conditions, seek help from a nutritional therapist who can help you make better progress. A review of your medication can be organised by your GP, so let him or her know your concerns.

Constant stress

We have explored in earlier chapters the effects of stress on the body and the immune system, and on pain. Stress contributes substantially to the onset and progression of arthritis. If you were to follow all the recommendations made within this book, without changing anything to do with your stress, your arthritis would improve, but only to a point. Your recovery will be hampered by this constant influence. First, look at whether or not stress can be reduced. In many cases it can, simply by taking the pressure off yourself and accepting you may have limitations for a while. On the other hand, however, the stress may be totally out of your control or unluckily, there will be one stress after another that makes your life difficult to cope with. Whatever is causing the stress, there are many nutrients that will support your body through the difficult times and protect your system from further damage. These nutrients include:

- B vitamins, especially B5 (pantothenic acid);
- vitamin C (in a buffered, non-acidic form such as calcium ascorbate);
- omega 3 (an essential fatty acid);
- theanine, an amino acid that induces a sense of calm. This tends to ensure you keep focus and will not make you feel drowsy;
- ginseng – all the varieties of ginseng have remarkable properties of supporting the adrenal glands (the glands most involved in the stress response of the body);
- ashwaghanda (*Withania somnifera*) – Indian ginseng. Helps the body adapt to a high level of stress. This herb is calming, nourishing and useful in cases where the person is very weak;
- passion flower (*passiflora*) – reduces anxiety and helps you to feel calm through stressful times;
- melissa (lemon balm);
- avena sativa (oats);
- St John's wort – this is a popular herb for alleviating mild anxiety and stress.

There are a few combination products available that are designed to support you through stressful periods. It may be appropriate to combine some of the above nutrients with simple lifestyle changes, such as taking up yoga or another calming activity; seeking help such as cognitive behavioural therapy; or devoting more time to relaxation, even if for only ten minutes a day. Regular practice of deep breathing exercises can also help your body to physically adapt to high stress.

Poor diet

There is a great deal of dietary advice in this book. However, it may not be possible to follow it due to your situation. If so, use treatment plan 2 on page 77 (for those who are unable to prepare food adequately) for guidance, as you may need to take extra supplements to counteract your poor quality food intake. The situation will improve as you progress and your capabilities return, enabling you to prepare and cook more appropriate foods for your health.

Sleeping difficulties

Sleep gives your body the opportunity to rest, relax and repair itself. While you are asleep, your body is trying very hard to heal any damage it has sustained and help you recover from the day's events. Many people have sleeping problems, ranging from mild restlessness to extreme insomnia. This may be due to stress, hormonal imbalance, blood sugar imbalances, spending too much time on a computer or watching television, lack of exercise, night-time disturbances and noise, light in the bedroom, or pain from your condition. Once you have given it all the nutrients from the day's food and supplement intake, your body needs time to assimilate them and put them to good use. Sleep is the opportunity to achieve this. If sleep is prevented or impaired, the progress of your treatment may be affected. The following steps can be taken to ensure a better night's sleep:

- Do not drink tea, coffee or any foods containing caffeine after 4 p.m.
- Do not eat a large meal late at night. Your body will be focused on digesting rather than sleeping.
- Ensure that the room you sleep in is dark. Buy blackout blinds and make sure there are no lights from any sources within the room. Melatonin, the hormone responsible for sending you to sleep, is responsive to light and dark and may not be active if the room is still light.
- Electromagnetic radiation from sources such as computers, televisions,

refrigerators, microwaves, etc., interferes with the body's production of melatonin, the sleep hormone. Spending fewer hours each day in close proximity to these electrical devices, particularly later in the day, may help improve sleep patterns.

- Try breathing exercises or listening to relaxing music quietly before bedtime. This helps prepare your body for sleep.
- Take an Epsom salts bath if possible. This provides magnesium, the mineral that helps calm the nervous system and induce sleep. If a bath is impossible, do the next best thing: spray your body with magnesium oil.
- You may need the help of supplements. Choose from the following: valerian, hops, amino acids 5-HTP (this turns into melatonin in the body), L-theanine, vitamin B6 or homeopathic remedies – these are particularly useful if you are losing sleep due to stress or anxiety.

Lack of compliance

This is another way of simply saying human nature. There will be many occasions when you feel you can't follow the diet or you forget to take the supplements or baths. First, don't be too hard on yourself. Second, try again. Unfortunately your health problems aren't going to vanish and they will still be there tomorrow. Tackling them head-on and with perseverance is the only way of overcoming your problems once and for all.

The other aspect of this issue is thinking that nutritional supplements are simply naturally sourced pharmaceutical drugs. The truth is that if you take nutrition in the same way that you take pharmaceutical drugs – swallow pills, drugs or otherwise – and don't address dietary factors such as diet and any others involved in your particular situation, then success is rare. Why is this? There are several issues that affect how natural supplements work:

- The dose may not be adequate; label instructions are often conservative and the advice on dose is often (although not always) higher when you are under professional supervision.
- You may need nutrient co-factors, such as a particular mineral, to ensure proper absorption.
- By taking just one nutrient you may upset the balance of other nutrients. Nutrients tend to work synergistically in the body. For example, calcium and magnesium pair up in their actions and if you were to

take a high amount or dose of calcium it might impair the levels and function of magnesium over a period of time.

- The time that you take your supplements can be crucial.
- A natural product may interfere with your medication, or may not be effective alongside it.
- You may need to make dietary changes to accompany your supplement plan for it to be effective.
- You may have an underlying issue that needs to be addressed differently for your recovery from arthritis to be sustained.

If none of the above help you and you are still struggling, you may need to seek the advice of a professional. This doesn't need to be expensive; often one visit can be enough to set you on the right track. However, it may be advisable to have a series of sessions over a period of time to ensure that your progress is as expected. If you are concerned about the cost, financial limits can be discussed beforehand, as there may be different options available to obtain the advice you need. Making an enquiry doesn't cost a penny.

If you decide to consult a nutritional therapy practitioner, he or she will have access to specialist supplements and will be able to advise you exactly what to take, how many to take, at what time of day and so on, to get the best results. Your therapist will also identify any underlying health problems that may be affecting you and gradually you will work together until you achieve a sustainable outcome: NO pain, NO stiffness and NO feelings of weakness or ill-health whatsoever.

10

Testimonials

At the Margaret Hills Clinic, we have many positive accounts of people who have recovered completely from their arthritis by following our guidance. Still a family business, now in its third generation, we are here to support you through your treatment and ensure you have the confidence to pursue your recovery. Here are just a few testimonials, written by the patients themselves (their names have been changed to maintain their anonymity).

First is Roberta, who was reluctant to use conventional treatment for her osteoarthritis due to past experiences of close family with the condition:

Roberta

At the age of 49 I developed osteoarthritis in my toe joints. This became so painful that I had to wear special shoes to enable me to work, my limping became worse and it was more painful at night – rather oddly – when the throbbing pain kept me awake – I felt 149 years old!

My doctor advised steroid injections but I had none – thank God. What had that done for my mother and my grandfather when they were pumped full of drugs? I resolved never to go down that route, unless I was absolutely desperate.

Within 9 months (of natural treatment) I began to feel less pain and after a year and a half I was back in my normal shoes again and with just the odd bad day.

After two and a half years all pain had gone and now after five years the swelling on my joints, including my distorted finger joints has subsided . . . I only wish I could have saved my mother the agony she endured . . .

The only vinegar I take is organic cider vinegar, which I actually now quite enjoy despite my earlier reservations!

Yvonne came to us with polymyalgia rheumatica, an inflammatory rheumatic condition affecting the muscles rather than the joints (the term 'polymyalgia' means 'many painful/aching muscles'). She attributes her recovery to diet and a positive state of mind:

Yvonne

My doctor was so pleased with my progress re PMR (polymyalgia rheumatica) that he said he need not see me again. I put this down to diet etc., encouragement and some prayer.

My blood tests have been good for some time, ESR [erythrocyte sedimentation rate, which measures the level of infection and inflammation] low and stable, zinc test still positive. I feel fine and people comment on how well I look, also I have not had any arthritic pain for what seems like years.

Geoff, who we also treated for polymyalgia rheumatica, made an equally successful recovery after four years:

Geoff

In March 1991 I contracted polymyalgia rheumatica – acute muscle pain. The immediate treatment was 30 mg of Prednisolone and 100 mg of Voltarol (non-steroid painkiller). My GP was giving me weekly examinations and keeping a check on blood pressure and my eyes. I had seen the rheumatoid arthritis specialist who said, 'The good news is that this illness can burn itself out in anything up to ten years – the bad news is that the dose of steroid you must take to avoid blindness may cause side effects, but we can treat osteoporosis.' I was depressed. In fact, PMR brings about depression.

I knew about the Margaret Hills Clinic, using drug-free methods to treat rheumatoid and osteoarthritis, and I visited. The programme was to build the immune system, not suppress it. The regime included supplements such as zinc and a formula rich in vitamins, DLPA (an essential amino acid), alfalfa, cider vinegar and honey.

In two months my ESR was down to 21, from 97. In the next month it reduced to 4 and two weeks later it was 0. It took about seven months for me to gradually come off the steroid and Voltarol, against my GP's advice.

It took four years for me to be free of PMR. But I know that the Margaret Hills regime allowed me to be free of further side effects. Other patients (who don't know of the Margaret Hills Clinic) continue to use the steroids and Voltarol. They cannot reduce the steroid beyond 5 mg a day and are risking illnesses such as rheumatoid arthritis and possibly osteoporosis as side effects of the steroid treatment. Nothing is prescribed for patients to relieve the depression which accompanies the disease.

Josephine, meanwhile, had been diagnosed with rheumatoid arthritis and osteoarthritis:

Josephine

It is now nearly a year since I contacted the Margaret Hills Clinic in some degree of desperation following the onset of both rheumatoid arthritis and osteoarthritis.

Confronted with a future full of pain and restricted movement, the strength in my hands had become greatly diminished and my fingers were swollen. I was very stiff; after sitting in a chair for 30 minutes I had difficulty getting up.

I started upon the Margaret Hills acid free diet in August 2006. After a few weeks the swelling in my fingers became diminished and the pain began to fade; by Christmas 2006 I was pain free throughout my body. I have no stiffness at all.

It is not an easy road to go down, it is a tough regime but the reward is enormous. I now lead a normal life, which includes an occasional glass of wine and a return to my beloved yoga class.

I feel like I have escaped a prison sentence.

Diana gives a detailed account of recovery from severe rheumatoid arthritis, during which time other health problems also disappeared:

Diana

Officially in December 2008 I was diagnosed with rheumatoid arthritis. I had excruciating pain in my left wrist which was swollen.

I refused all the medication my doctor offered me. I was told if I did not take the medication I would be a cripple in three months' time. I still refused and he told me if I changed my mind in six months' time he would still treat me.

As I was already doing the cider vinegar treatment, after my husband found the Margaret Hills Clinic on the internet, I started the full treatment with the formula just before Christmas 2008.

By that time it had got so bad that:

- I could no longer hold a knife or lift anything in the kitchen.
- I had to be helped on/off the toilet.
- I could not turn around in bed on my own.
- I had to be helped on and off a chair.
- I walked with a stoop.
- I could not dress myself or do up any buttons.
- My legs and feet were swollen and shoes did not fit me.

From one day to the next I could not write my name on a cheque – it looked like the scribble of a two year old.

I was in a desperate state and very, very down. Not at all like me.

I changed my diet overnight: not a good idea. Then with the help of the Margaret Hills Clinic I got myself sorted, but it took a long, long time. After a month of the treatment I started to feel better.

I am now on three capsules a day (of natural vitamins and minerals) and one cider vinegar drink a day (for life) and am happy to do so.

I walk tall and am fit and healthy thanks to the treatment. It took me just over a year to rid myself of the arthritis. And if I can do it, so can anybody else. There is no quick fix, but it works.

I am very grateful to the team at the Clinic, without them I would not be where I am today, without pain. And I will never, never allow myself to get to the state of that excruciating pain ever again.

Before I started on the treatment I did take medication:

- warfarin for palpitations 7 mg (4 years)
- Symbicort for asthma (3 years)
- Bricanyl for asthma (3 years)

Now I take nothing at all, thanks to the treatment.

It was a long struggle but I have made it. I do sometimes treat myself to a bacon sandwich. But that's about all. I will always do the diet.

Finally, here is a copy of a letter from a consultant rheumatologist to one of his patients indicating the shortcomings of conventional treatment:

Dear George,

I was sorry to hear that you had a nasty reaction to Salazopyrin. This is pretty rare but it really means that we cannot put you back on Salazopyrin.

To date you have tried all of the commonly used drugs for the treatment of arthritis.

There are a couple of options here:

• The first is simply to take a holiday from drugs and see how your arthritis behaves on its own over the next few months.

• You could also see what alternative medicine has to offer.

• There are a few other drugs which could be used but I am not optimistic that they are going to work for you. You have been very unlucky with medications to date and it may simply be that the risks of medications for you outweigh the benefits.

If you want a further appointment to discuss further treatment options, please ring.

Yours sincerely

This letter paints a picture of the typical situation that leads to people searching for alternative treatments. Although this case is of someone who experienced very severe reactions, many people more commonly suffer from side effects that are troublesome enough to warrant different treatment options.

11

Prevention is better then cure

This book has mainly been written for people who already have arthritis. Nevertheless, the advice it contains is also valuable if you do not have arthritis yet. There's plenty you can do to reduce the chances of developing arthritis; don't sit back and wait for it to affect you, or until you are experiencing more than just a few niggles.

If you don't have arthritis at the moment, you may be prone to developing the condition at a later date if you:

- are aged over 50;
- have a higher than normal amount of stress in your life;
- have had a consistently poor diet of processed foods with inadequate nutrients up to now;
- have relatives who have arthritis of any type;
- have minor aches and pains; or
- undertake sports and fitness activities regularly.

Act now to prevent arthritis from affecting you. Follow the guidelines of the alkaline diet and perhaps take a once-weekly Epsom salts bath, together with cider vinegar drinks daily. Small, simple measures such as these are easy to implement and may well prevent the onset of any type of arthritis, not to mention other health problems.

Medical health professionals are trained in the treatment and care management of existing conditions. Little emphasis is placed on the prevention techniques necessary to reduce the likelihood or severity of arthritis. In fact, you may not even be offered a referral to a specialist consultant until your symptoms progress to a more extreme level. People with arthritis are often expected to go home and use paracetamol or an anti-inflammatory drug if they need to and wait it out until the severity of their symptoms becomes more difficult to control.

Only at this stage will their future treatment options be discussed. In most cases, this means stronger types of drugs, associated with more side effects, to help them while they wait for an operation to replace the affected joint.

Unfortunately this tends to be the way of modern healthcare systems, but you don't need to wait for this to happen to you. Acting early to overcome symptoms will help you avoid the inevitability of worsening arthritis. Health professionals will help to guide you on to the right path, but ultimately taking charge of your own condition and acting positively to overcome it is the best possible solution.

This book focuses on the treatment and management of arthritis. From a naturopathic viewpoint, however, I must emphasize the importance of prevention. Most cases of chronic arthritis can be prevented if, as an individual, you prioritize your own health via dietary means, physical exercise, fresh air and a calm mind. Learn to listen to your body – prevention is far easier to achieve than cure.

Useful addresses

Margaret Hills Clinic
1 Oaks Precinct
Caesar Road
Kenilworth
Warwickshire CV8 1DP
Tel.: 01926 854783
Website: www.margarethillsclinic.com

Margaret Hills Health and Lifestyle
Unit 7, Millar Court
43 Station Road
Kenilworth
Warwickshire CV8 1JD
Tel.: 01926 850019
Website: www.margarethillsclinic.com

Riverford Organic Vegetables Ltd
Wash Farm
Buckfastleigh
Devon TQ11 0JU
Tel.: 01803 762059
Website: www.riverford.co.uk

This firm operates a vegetable-box delivery scheme throughout the UK. There are four farms which make up Riverford. The box scheme started in the registered office at the address above. There are three others: Riverford on Sacrewell Farm near Peterborough; Riverford on Home Farm in Yorkshire; Riverford on Upper Norton Farm in Hampshire. Vegetables are grown and delivered by the farm that is regional to your own particular address.

If you are seeking tests for food allergies and intolerances, the following organization will be able to help:

YorkTest Laboratories Ltd
York Science Park
York YO10 5DQ
Tel.: 01904 410410; 0800 074 6185 (freephone – UK only)
Website: www.yorktest.com

References

Introduction

1 Schmitz, N., Kraus, V. B., Aigner, T. 'Targets to tackle – the pathophysiology of the disease', *Current Drug Targets* 11:5 (May 2010), 521–7

1 What is arthritis and what might cause it?

1 Schmitz, N., Kraus, V. B., Aigner, T. 'Targets to tackle – the pathophysiology of the disease', *Current Drug Targets* 11:5 (May 2010), 521–7
2 Farwell, W., Taylor, E. 'Serum anion gap, bicarbonate and biomarkers of inflammation in healthy individuals in a national survey', *Canadian Medical Association Journal* 182:2 (February 2010), 137–41

2 Natural treatment for arthritis: the three-category principle

1 British Medical Association & Royal Pharmaceutical Society of Great Britain. *British National Formulary*, BMJ Publishing Group Ltd, London & RPS Publishing, London. September 2007

3 Category 1: alkalizing the body

1 Pattison, D., Symmons, D., Young, A. 'Does diet have a role in the aetiology of rheumatoid arthritis?', *Proceedings of the Nutrition Society* 63 (2004), 137–43
2 Hung Ro Kim et al. 'Nutrition and disease – green tea protects rats against autoimmune arthritis by modulating disease-related immune events', *Journal of Nutrition* 138:11 (November 2008), 2111–16
3 Rubin, J. 'Attacking the seven causes of inflammation', *Townsend Letter* (Feb/Mar 2003), 111–14
4 Van der Kraan, P., et al. 'High susceptibility of human articular cartilage glycosaminoglycan synthesis to changes in inorganic sulfate availability', *Journal of Orthopaedic Research* 8:4 (July 1990), 565–71
5 Benedetti, S., et al. 'Biomarkers of oxidation, inflammation and cartilage degradation in osteoarthritis patients undergoing sulfur-based spa therapies', *Clinical Biochemistry* 43:12 (August 2010), 973–8
6 Rizzo, R., Grandolfo, M., et al. 'Calcium, sulfur, and zinc distribution in normal and arthritic articular equine cartilage: a synchrotron radiation-induced X-ray emission (SRIXE) study', *Journal of Experimental Zoology* 273:1 (September 1995), 82–6

7   Kim, L. S., Axelrod, L. J., Howard, P., et al. 'Efficacy of MSM in osteoarthritis pain of the knee: a pilot clinical trial', *Osteoarthritis Cartilage* 14:3 (2006), 286–94
8   Reyed, R. M., El-Diwany, A. 'Molasses as bifidus promoter on bifidobacteria and lactic acid bacteria growing in skim milk', *The Internet Journal of Microbiology* 5:1 (2008)
9   Nenonen, M. T., et al. 'Uncooked, lactobacilli-rich, vegan food and rheumatoid arthritis', *Rheumatology* 37:3 (1998), 274–81

4 Category 2: joint repair nutrients

1   Chaganti, R. K., Parimi, N., Cawthon P. 'Association of 25-hydroxyvitamin D with prevalent osteoarthritis of the hip in elderly men: The osteoporotic fractures in men study', *Arthritis & Rheumatism* 62:2 (February 2010), 511–14
2   Adorini, L. 'Treatment of immunomediated diseases by vitamin D analogs', *Nutrition and Health* 7 (2010), 1025–41
3   Rousseau, J. C., Delmas, P. 'Biological markers in osteoarthritis', *Nature Clinical Practice Rheumatology* 3 (March 2007), 346–56
4   Mohammad Shahi, M., Mahboub, S. A., et al. 'Effect of isolated soy protein on prevention of rheumatoid arthritis in collagen-induced rats', *QOM University of Medical Sciences Journal* 3:1 (2009), 1–12
5   Volpi, N. 'The pathobiology of osteoarthritis and the rationale for using the chondroitin sulfate for its treatment', *Current Drug Targets Immune, Endocrine and Metabolic Disorders* 4:2 (2004), 119–27
6   Uebelhart, D. 'Clinical review of chondroitin sulfate in osteoarthritis', *Osteoarthritis Cartilage* 16 Suppl. 3 (2008), 19–21
7   Matsuno, H., et al. 'Effects of an oral administration of glucosamine-chondroitin-quercetin glucoside on the synovial fluid properties in patients with osteoarthritis and rheumatoid arthritis', *Bioscience, Biotechnology, and Biochemistry* 73 (2009), 288–92
8   Kubo, M., Ando, K., et al. 'Chondroitin sulfate for the treatment of hip and knee osteoarthritis: Current status and future trends', *Life Sciences* 85:13–14 (September 2009), 477–83
9   Qiu, G. X., Gao, S. N., et al. 'Efficacy and safety of glucosamine sulfate versus ibuprofen in patients with knee osteoarthritis', *Arzneimittelforschung/Drug Research* 48:5 (June 1998), 469–74
10 Theiler, R., Bruhlmann, P. 'Overall tolerability and analgesic activity of intraarticular sodium hyaluronate in the treatment of knee osteoarthritis', *Current Medical Research and Opinion* 21:11 (November 2005), 1727–33
11 Neustadt, D., Caldwell, J., et al. 'Clinical effects of intraarticular injection of high molecular weight hyaluronan (Orthovisc) in osteoarthritis of the knee: a randomized, controlled, multicenter trial', *Journal of Rheumatology* 32:10 (October 2005), 1928–36; Huang, M. H., Yang, R. C., et al. 'Preliminary results of integrated therapy for patients with knee osteoarthritis', *Arthritis and Rheumatism* 53:6 (December 2005), 812–20

5 Category 3: supplements to relieve inflammation and pain

1 Chaitow, L. *Amino Acids in Therapy*. Wellingborough: Thorsons, p. 59

2 Fox, A., Fox, B. *DLPA: The Natural Painkiller and Antidepressant*. Wellingborough: Thorsons, 1987

3 Greenwald, R. A., 'Oxygen radicals, inflammation, and arthritis: Pathophysiological considerations and implications for treatment', *Seminars in Arthritis and Rheumatism* 20:4 (February 1991), 219–40

4 Regan, E., Flannelly, J., et al. 'Extracellular superoxide dismutase and oxidant damage in osteoarthritis', *Arthritis and Rheumatism* 52:11 (November 2005), 3479–91

5 Choi, E. J., Bae, S. C., et al. 'Dietary vitamin E and quercetin modulate inflammatory responses of collagen-induced arthritis in mice', *Journal of Medicinal Food* 12:4 (August 2009), 770–5

6 Mcalindon, T. E., et al. 'Do antioxidant micronutrients protect against the development and progression of knee osteoarthritis?', *Arthritis and Rheumatism* 39:4 (April 1996), 648–56

7 Feinstein, A. *Healing with Vitamins*. Emmaus, PA: Rodale Books, 1996

8 Heliövaara, M., Knekt, P., et al. 'Serum antioxidants and risk of rheumatoid arthritis', *Annals of the Rheumatic Diseases* 53 (1994), 51–3

9 Cho, M. L., Heo, Y. J., et al. 'Grape seed proanthocyanidin extract (GSPE) attenuates collagen-induced arthritis', *Immunology Letters* 124:2 (June 2009), 102–10

10 Bauerova, K., Paulovicova, E., et al. 'Combined methotrexate and coenzyme Q(10) therapy in adjuvant-induced arthritis evaluated using parameters of inflammation and oxidative stress', *The Journal of the Polish Biochemical Society* 57:3 (2010), 347–54

11 Havsteen, B. 'Flavonoids, a class of natural products of high pharmacological potency', *Biochemical Pharmacology* 32:7 (1983), 1141–8

12 Akhtar, N. M., Naseer, R., et al. 'Oral enzyme combination versus diclofenac in the treatment of osteoarthritis of the knee – a double-blind prospective randomized study', *Journal of Clinical Rheumatology* 23:5 (October 2004), 410–15

13 Hurst, S., Zainal, Z., et al. 'Dietary fatty acids and arthritis', *Prostaglandins, Leukotrienes and Essential Fatty Acids* 82:4 (April 2010), 315–18

14 Rennie, K. L., Hughes, J., et al. 'Nutritional management of rheumatoid arthritis: a review of the evidence', *Journal of Human Nutrition and Diet* 16:2 (April 2003), 97–109

15 Kremer, J. M., Lawrence, D. A., et al. 'Effects of high-dose fish oil on rheumatoid arthritis after stopping nonsteroidal anti-inflammatory drugs. Clinical and immune correlates', *Arthritis and Rheumatism* 38:8 (August 1995), 1107–14

16 Akram, M., Ibrahim Shah, M., et al. '*Zingiber officinale* Roscoe (a medicinal plant)', *Pakistan Journal of Nutrition* 10:4 (2011), 399–400

17 Owais, M. 'Clinical evaluation of herbal medicine for the treatment of

rheumatoid arthritis', M. Phil thesis, Hamdard University, Karachi (2009)

18 Altman, R. D., Marcussen, K. C. 'Effects of a ginger extract on knee pain in patients with osteoarthritis', *Arthritis and Rheumatism* 44:11 (November 2001), 2531–8

19 Grzanna, R., Lindmark, L., Frondoza, C. G. 'Ginger – an herbal medicinal product with broad anti-inflammatory actions', *Journal of Medicinal Food* 8:2 (2005), 125–32

20 Srivastava, K. C., Mustafa, T. 'Ginger (*Zingiber officinale*) in rheumatism and musculoskeletal disorders', *Medical Hypotheses* 39 (1992), 342–9

21 Joe, B., Lokesh, B. R. 'Effect of curcumin and capsaicin on arachidonic acid metabolism and lysosomal enzyme secretion by rat peritoneal macrophages', *Lipids* 32:11 (December 1997), 1173–80

22 Etzel, R. 'Special extract of Boswellia Serrata (H17) in the treatment of rheumatoid arthritis', *Phytomedicine* 3 (1996), 91–4

23 Singh, G. B., Bani, S., Singh, S. 'Toxicity and safety evaluation of boswellic acids', *Phytomedicine* 3 (1996), 87–90

24 Warnock, M., McBean, D., et al. 'Effectiveness and safety of Devil's Claw tablets in patients with general rheumatic disorders', *Phytotherapy Research* 21:12 (December 2007), 1228–33

7 Putting it all together

1 Fletcher, R. H., Fairfield, K. M. 'Vitamins for chronic disease prevention in adults: clinical applications', *Journal of the American Medical Association* 287:23 (19 June 2002), 3127–9

8 Exercise and joint health

1 Percival, M. 'Nutritional support for connective tissue repair and wound healing', *Clinical Nutrition Insights* (1997), 1–5. Available at <http://acudoc.com/Injury%20Healing.PDF>

Index

The main entries are shown in bold print.